Super Easy Anti-Inflammatory Cookbook for Beginners

CALLIE PEAY

TABLE OF CONTENTS

Introduction

If your joints, muscles, or tendons suffer when you move, anti-inflammatory medicine is the solution. Anti-inflammatories are becoming more common as people become more active to combat conditions such as osteoarthritis and carpal tunnel syndrome, whether it's taking corticosteroids (as prescribed by your doctor), using an over-the-counter cold remedy containing ibuprofen, or adopting a healthier diet, such as substituting fresh fruit and vegetables for processed foods. However, some physicians prescribe them for migraine headaches that are aggravated by strenuous exercise.

Consume more healthful meals to reduce inflammation. Try to eat a variety of meals that are abundant in nutrients, healthy fats, and antioxidants. This is the anti-inflammatory diet philosophy in a nutshell.

Some foods increase inflammation, while others assist to alleviate it. In the anti-inflammatory diet, processed foods, foods with added sugar, red meats, and alcohol are avoided or prohibited. Fruits and vegetables, omega-3 fatty acid-rich meals, whole grains, lean protein, healthy fats, and spices are preferred instead. These anti-inflammatory foods are high in antioxidants, which aid the body in ridding itself of free radicals. Our systems create antioxidants to aid in the removal of free radicals; but they sometimes need the support of dietary antioxidants as well. Although free radicals are produced as a result of some activities, such as metabolism, their levels in the body may be elevated by external irritants such as stress or bad food.

I welcome you to give a review on this book after you have finished reading it. This would mean a lot to me since it would help spread the word about this material; you know I worked extremely hard on this product, and I truly hope you love it!

The Advantages of an Anti-Inflammatory Diet

Anti-Inflammatory Diet Principles

Consume less sugar: This is important to remember. When I mention "sugar," I'm not only referring to table sugar. Refined carbs are turned to sugar in the body. Refined carbs include white bread, white rice, and French fries. The American Heart Association (2018) recommends that males eat roughly nine teaspoons of sugar per day, while women consume approximately six teaspoons. I know chocolate and sweets are appealing, but we must resist and go for fruit instead.
Reduce your dairy consumption: While fermented dairy products, such as yogurt, are generally safe to ingest, fresh dairy products might induce inflammation on occasion.
Consume an abundance of fresh fruits and vegetables: These are high in antioxidants, as well as vitamins and fiber.
Eat omega-3-rich meals like fish: This fatty acid is often lacking in our diet. We obtain a lot of Omega-6 from vegetable oils and processed meals, but it must be balanced with Omega-3.
Avoid processed foods: The anti-inflammatory diet focuses on eating fresh, natural foods. I think we can all agree that processed foods are detrimental to our health. Meal planning can help you avoid these meals significantly.
The diet is all about packing your meals with foods that may help you combat inflammation. You will also need to eliminate any foods that lead to inflammation. The anti-inflammatory diet is more of a way of life than a diet. It is a diet that aids in the reduction of low-grade inflammation in the body. Ideally, you should eat more vegetables and fruits every day, restrict your intake of dairy and red meat, choose complex carbohydrates, and avoid processed foods. You'll also need to eat omega-3-rich meals like anchovies, salmon, mussels, and halibut.

The Strategy for Getting the Most Out of Your Anti-Inflammatory Diet

1. Fiber should be a key component of your anti-inflammatory diet strategy.
Fiber is beneficial to intestinal health. Fiber in the diet is also crucial for maintaining normal blood glucose levels. It also enhances the body's insulin sensitivity.

2. Nutrient supplements must include fruits and vegetables.
Those in quest of the greatest vitamin supplements have every reason to quit up. The bulk of the nutrients required for a healthy body and mind are found in fruits and vegetables. They include a lot of vitamins, minerals, and antioxidants. They are simple to digest and help to reduce inflammation.
Every day, you should eat at least 4-5 servings of fruits and vegetables. Leafy greens, cruciferous vegetables, and fruits are all anti-inflammatory foods. Your anti-inflammatory diet will be

inefficient and unsuccessful if you exclude them. They spice up your life and make you seem as healthy and active as they do.

3. Crucifers, in combination with onion, ginger, and garlic, may be very beneficial to your health. It is common knowledge that cruciferous vegetables such as broccoli, cauliflower, and Brussels sprouts are abundant in nutrients. Their anti-inflammatory capabilities are quite strong. Add ginger, garlic, and onion to your recipes to increase their intensity and taste. They collaborate to fortify your immune system. Flavor may also be added to your foods by using onion, ginger, and garlic. For taste, you may also experiment with additional spices.

4. Consumption of more than 10% saturated fat might be harmful.
Saturated fats are bad for your health. They may increase the risk of heart disease and trigger the production of free radicals. Consuming more than 20 grams of saturated fat per 2000 calories per day is not recommended.
Consumption of red meat must be minimized. It is tough to digest and contains a lot of fat. To prevent the development of harmful chemicals while cooking, marinate it with herbs, spices, vinegar, and fresh fruit juices before eating.

5. Omega-3 fatty acids are quite important.
Fruits, vegetables, shellfish, and nuts are high in omega-3 fatty acids. You must eat enough of these things on a daily basis. Omega-3 fatty acids are essential for decreasing inflammation and the risk of chronic inflammation-related illnesses. Cancer, arthritis, heart disease, and neurological disorders are just a few of the illnesses that ingesting omega-3 fatty acids might help you prevent.

6. Increase your intake of cold-water seafood.
Omega-3 fatty acids are abundant in wild cold water fish such as salmon, mackerel, and trout. They also include the bulk of the other vitamins and minerals required. Consuming this sort of fish on a daily or weekly basis can considerably improve your immunity. These fish provide all of the antioxidants needed for an anti-inflammatory diet. If you don't want to consume fish or can't get wild-caught cold-water fish, molecularly distilled fish oil pills are one option. It would be a shame to miss out on any of the alternatives.

7. Use healthy oils for the greatest outcomes.
Food may look incomplete without oils and fat, but choosing the wrong oil might cost you a lot of money. Bad oil may hurt your heart and boost free radical production. Your body needs fat, but it does not have to be harmful fat.
There are several healthy oil choices, such as virgin and extra virgin olive oil. You may also use expeller pressed canola or sunflower oil. Polyphenols, which serve as antioxidants, are abundant in these.

8. Use fruits and spices to add flavor to your dishes.

It is vital to recognize that if you do not practice self-control, all of your efforts will be futile. Taste is an essential part of life; without it, everything might become boring. However, looking for it in refined sugar and artificial sweeteners might be a major mistake. These goods not only increase fructose buildup, but they may also raise insulin resistance and the risk of type 2 diabetes.
Fruits are naturally occurring sugar alternatives. The sugar component of the fruits will help to regulate blood sugar, and the digestive fiber will absorb any excess glucose. Fruits may improve your health while adding taste to your meals. Spices are another technique to flavor foods.

9. One or two servings of beans and legumes each day will go you far.
When most veggies are overdone, they lose nutrients. Beans and legumes, however, do not come within this group. They are versatile and rich in minerals, protein, and soluble fiber. Furthermore, they are both pleasant and healthful. If you exclude them from your daily anti-inflammatory diet, you will become deficient.
Physical exercise is also important.
The value of physical exercise in your anti-inflammatory diet is something you should never overlook. Physical exercise boosts your immune system and aids your body in its battle against inflammation. Your body can absorb nutrients more quickly and battle chronic ailments more effectively. Even tiny amounts of physical exercise, such as a brisk stroll, may aid in hormone regulation and maintaining a healthy balance. You will feel more revitalized and renewed.

The Benefits of an Anti-Inflammatory Diet

An anti-inflammatory diet is beneficial to our health. Anti-inflammatory foods are abundant in antioxidants and vitamins, which help to reduce inflammation.
An anti-inflammatory diet is not a new idea; it has been around for quite some time. Many individuals have tried and had excellent success with it. It may surprise you to find that your favorite food might induce inflammation in your body.
An anti-inflammatory diet is good for your heart. Northwestern University research found that omega-3 fatty acid-rich foods including fish, nuts, and plants may help protect the cardiovascular system against inflammation. Eating fish twice a week may thereby reduce the chance of acquiring heart disease by half.
An anti-inflammatory diet will improve your joints in the following ways: Anti-inflammatory foods may lower your chances of developing osteoporosis by preserving your joints. The rationale is that omega-3 fatty acids may aid in the health and strength of your bones. Furthermore, anti-inflammatory diets, according to the National Osteoporosis Foundation, include antioxidants that may assist in the battle against this disorder.
Your gut will benefit from an anti-inflammatory diet: "Why does my stomach hurt?" is a frequently asked question. Foods rich in fiber and anti-inflammatory compounds, such as fruits, vegetables, and whole grains, may help reduce irritable bowel syndrome (IBS).

Following an anti-inflammatory diet may assist you in avoiding obesity. Overeating, which may contribute to fat tissue development and obesity, is discouraged in this approach.

Obesity and an inflammatory diet may be linked in many ways. One inflammatory diet includes eating more refined carbs, processed meats, and junk food. Due to the low calorie and fiber content of these meals, a person will need to eat more to compensate for the calorie shortfall and lack of satisfaction. People who eat an inflammatory diet may spend more time inside, which encourages them to consume more calories while exercising less.

People who already have inflammatory problems may benefit the most from an anti-inflammatory diet. Diets high in refined sugars and carbs have been linked to type 2 diabetes, metabolic syndrome, and obesity. Instead, an anti-inflammatory diet recommends consuming whole grains such as brown rice, which is rich in fiber and has a low glycemic index.

A low-inflammatory diet may also help with weariness. The presence of inflammation suggests that the immune system is working appropriately. Histamine levels increase when the immune system is entirely devoted, making a person drowsy, lethargic, and grumpy. The operations of the immune system are designed to make you fatigued, enabling your body to slow down and preserve energy. Fatigue is also regarded to encourage rest and healing rather than further restricting the body. An anti-inflammatory diet helps to minimize or eliminate inflammation, which lessens or eliminates the immune system's fatigue-causing effects.

Weight reduction may be aided by an anti-inflammatory diet that has nothing to do with obesity. You may be overweight or on the edge of being fat even if you are not obese. The excessive intake of refined carbohydrates and sugars is blamed for accidental weight gain as well as other non-dietary factors such as sedentary lifestyles. Refined carbohydrate diets are deficient in nutrients and so need more calories than necessary.

An anti-inflammatory diet may help you sleep better. In a number of ways, diet may contribute to poor sleep quality or an erratic sleep pattern. When you consume an inflammatory diet, you will have trouble sleeping on a regular basis, and the sleep you do get will be of poor quality. An inflammatory diet may lead to eating problems, such as waking up in the middle of the night to eat, which can interfere with the quality and duration of sleep. You may need repeated periods of short sleeping due to weariness, which will interrupt your night's sleep. An anti-inflammatory diet, on the other hand, may help you sleep better by decreasing inflammation and ensuring that your meals are calorie and mineral balanced.

The most significant advantage of adopting an anti-inflammatory diet is that it may significantly lower your risk of heart disease. People who eat an anti-inflammatory diet are much less likely to acquire heart disease than those who do not. Why is this the case? An anti-inflammatory diet, on the other hand, aids in the reduction of inflammation in the body, which has been connected to the development of heart disease.

Foods to Eat

- Dark leafy greens such as kale and spinach
- Blackberries, blueberries, and cherries
- Grapes

- Cauliflower and broccoli
- Grass tea
- Beans and lentils
- Coconut and avocado
- Olives
- Olive oil
- Nuts such as walnuts, almonds, pistachios, pine nuts, and others
- Cold water fish (and other types of fish as well) such as salmon and sardines
- Cinnamon, turmeric, and other spices

Red meat is a significant generator of inflammation in the body. It has been shown to raise three blood indicators linked to heart disease and cancer. These include homocysteine, C-reactive protein (CRP), and lipoprotein.

Trans fats are associated with an increased risk of heart disease, stroke, diabetes, and inflammatory disorders including Crohn's and rheumatoid arthritis.

Whole milk: A research published in Nutrition Research found that consuming whole milk causes inflammation in overweight persons.

When the body is exposed to sugar, it might release more inflammatory proteins. This rise has been related to a wide range of health issues, including asthma, rheumatoid arthritis, and Alzheimer's disease.

Blue #1 and #2 dyes are often used in food items to enhance their vibrancy and attractiveness. Allergies, cancer, ADHD, and inflammation have all been related to the use of synthetic colors.

Caffeine is a natural stimulant that may boost energy, but it can also promote inflammation in the body.

Processed meats like bacon, sausage, and ham are usually heavy in salt and preservatives, both of which have been linked to inflammation.

Fast food, in particular, is heavy in added salt, sugar, and other chemicals that produce a lot of inflammation in the body.

Breakfast

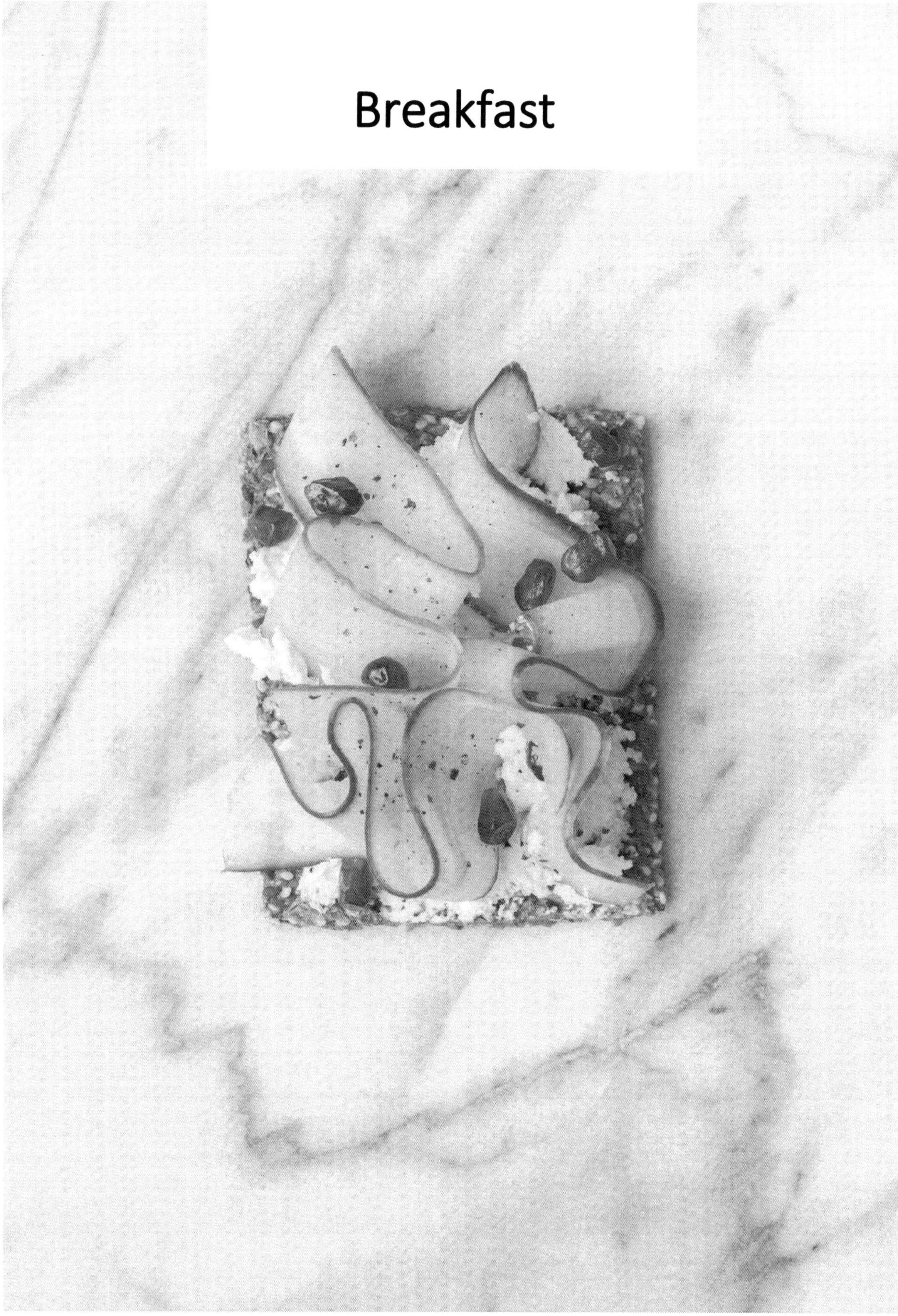

1. Avocado and Tomato Open Sandwich

Preparation Time: 10 minutes
Portion Size: 2

Ingredients:

4 slices whole grain bread
1 ripe avocado
1 ripe tomato, sliced
Salt and pepper to taste

Instructions:

Toast the bread slices.
Mash the avocado and spread evenly on the toast.
Top with tomato slices and season with salt and pepper.
Serve immediately.

Nutrition Facts (1 portion):

Energy: 290 Kcal
Carbs: 37 g
Proteins: 9 g
Fats: 13 g

2. Almond Milk Oatmeal

Preparation Time: 5 minutes
Cooking Time: 10 minutes
Portion Size: 2

Ingredients:

1 cup rolled oats
2 cups unsweetened almond milk
1 tbsp honey
1 cup mixed berries

Instructions:

Bring the almond milk to a boil in a pan.
Stir in the oats and reduce heat.
Simmer for 10 minutes, stirring occasionally.
Sweeten with honey and top with mixed berries.
Serve warm.

Nutrition Facts (1 portion):

Energy: 244 Kcal
Carbs: 42 g
Proteins: 7 g
Fats: 5 g

3. Pineapple Kale Smoothie

Preparation Time: 10 minutes
Portion Size: 2 servings

Ingredients:

1 cup fresh kale, de-stemmed
1 cup frozen pineapple chunks
1 ripe banana
1 cup unsweetened almond milk
1 tablespoon honey (optional)
Ice cubes (optional)

Instructions:

Place all the ingredients in a blender.
Blend on high speed until everything is smooth and well combined.
If the smoothie is too thick for your liking, you can add a little bit more almond milk or a few ice cubes and blend again.
Serve immediately in two glasses.

Nutrition Facts (1 portion):

Energy: 125 Kcal
Carbs: 30 g
Proteins: 3 g
Fats: 2 g

4. Tempeh and Veggie Stir-Fry

Preparation Time: 15 minutes
Cooking Time: 20 minutes
Portion Size: 2

Ingredients:

200g tempeh, cubed
1 bell pepper, sliced
1 medium carrot, sliced
1 zucchini, sliced
2 cloves garlic, minced
2 tablespoons tamari sauce
2 tablespoons olive oil
1 teaspoon ginger, minced

Instructions:

Heat the olive oil in a wok or large frying pan over medium heat.
Add the tempeh cubes and stir-fry until they are golden brown. Remove the tempeh from the pan and set aside.
In the same pan, add a little more oil if necessary, then add the garlic and ginger and stir-fry for about a minute.
Add the sliced vegetables and stir-fry until they are tender.
Return the tempeh to the pan, add the tamari sauce, and stir to combine.
Serve immediately with rice or noodles if desired.

Nutrition Facts (1 portion):

Energy: 350 Kcal
Carbs: 25 g
Proteins: 18 g
Fats: 20 g

5. Quinoa and Almond Porridge

Preparation Time: 5 minutes
Cooking Time: 15 minutes
Portion Size: 2

Ingredients:

1/2 cup quinoa
1 cup unsweetened almond milk
2 tbsp chopped almonds
1 tbsp honey

Instructions:

Rinse the quinoa and cook in almond milk according to package ***instructions***.
Allow to cool, then divide quinoa between two bowls.
Top with chopped almonds and drizzle with honey.
Serve warm.

Nutrition Facts (1 portion):

Energy: 258 Kcal
Carbs: 39 g
Proteins: 9 g
Fats: 8 g

6. Mango Chia Pudding

Preparation Time: 5 minutes
Resting Time: 4 hours
Portion Size: 2

Ingredients:

1 cup unsweetened almond milk
1/4 cup chia seeds
1 ripe mango, peeled and diced
1 tbsp honey

Instructions:

Combine almond milk and chia seeds in a bowl and stir well.

Cover and refrigerate for at least 4 hours, or until pudding consistency is reached.
Top with diced mango and drizzle with honey before serving.

Nutrition Facts (1 portion):
Energy: 260 Kcal
Carbs: 41 g
Proteins: 7 g
Fats: 9 g

7. Green Tea Smoothie

Preparation Time: 5 minutes
Portion Size: 2

Ingredients:
1 banana
1 cup spinach
1 cup brewed green tea, cooled
1 tbsp honey

Instructions:
Combine all ingredients in a blender and blend until smooth.
Serve immediately.

Nutrition Facts (1 portion):
Energy: 124 Kcal
Carbs: 32 g
Proteins: 2 g
Fats: 0 g

8. Baked Avocado Eggs

Preparation Time: 5 minutes
Cooking Time: 15 minutes
Portion Size: 2

Ingredients:
1 ripe avocado, halved and pitted
2 eggs
Salt and pepper to taste

Instructions:
Preheat oven to 425 degrees F.
Scoop out some of the avocado from the pitted area to create a well for the egg.
Crack an egg into each avocado half.
Season with salt and pepper.
Bake for 15 minutes, or until eggs are cooked to your liking.
Serve hot.

Nutrition Facts (1 portion):
Energy: 232 Kcal
Carbs: 9 g
Proteins: 7 g
Fats: 20 g

9. Cinnamon Apple Quinoa

Preparation Time: 5 minutes
Cooking Time: 15 minutes
Portion Size: 2

Ingredients:
1/2 cup quinoa
1 cup water
1 apple, diced
1 tsp cinnamon
2 tbsp honey

Instructions:
Rinse quinoa and cook in water according to package ***instructions***.
Stir in diced apple and cinnamon.
Serve hot, drizzled with honey.

Nutrition Facts (1 portion):
Energy: 279 Kcal
Carbs: 62 g

Proteins: 6 g
Fats: 2 g

10. Berry Greek Yogurt Parfait

Preparation Time: 10 minutes
Portion Size: 2

Ingredients:

2 cups low-fat Greek yogurt
1 cup mixed berries
2 tbsp honey
1/4 cup chopped almonds

Instructions:

In a glass, layer Greek yogurt, mixed berries, honey, and almonds.
Repeat the layers.
Serve immediately or refrigerate until serving.

Nutrition Facts (1 portion):

Energy: 215 Kcal
Carbs: 27 g
Proteins: 18 g
Fats: 5 g

11. Sweet Potato Hash

Preparation Time: 10 minutes
Cooking Time: 20 minutes
Portion Size: 2

Ingredients:

1 medium sweet potato, diced
1 small onion, diced
1 bell pepper, diced
2 eggs
1 tbsp olive oil
Salt and pepper to taste

Instructions:

Heat oil in a skillet over medium heat.
Add sweet potato, onion, and bell pepper, and sauté until soft and slightly browned.
Create wells in the hash and crack an egg into each.
Cover and cook until eggs are done to your liking.
Season with salt and pepper.
Serve hot.

Nutrition Facts (1 portion):

Energy: 245 Kcal
Carbs: 34 g
Proteins: 9 g
Fats: 9 g

12. Strawberry Banana Oatmeal

Preparation Time: 5 minutes
Cooking Time: 10 minutes
Portion Size: 2

Ingredients:

1 cup rolled oats
2 cups water
1 banana, sliced
1 cup strawberries, sliced
2 tbsp honey

Instructions:

Cook oats in water according to package ***instructions***.
Stir in sliced banana and strawberries.
Serve hot, sweetened with honey.

Nutrition Facts (1 portion):

Energy: 259 Kcal
Carbs: 60 g
Proteins: 6 g
Fats: 2 g

13. Spinach Banana Smoothie

Preparation Time: 5 minutes
Cooking Time: 0 minutes
Portion Size: 2

Ingredients:

1 banana
2 cups fresh spinach
1 cup almond milk (unsweetened)
1 tablespoon honey

Instructions:

Combine banana, spinach, almond milk, and honey in a blender.
Blend until smooth and creamy.
Serve immediately, preferably chilled.

Nutrition Facts (1 portion):

Energy: 150 Kcal
Carbs: 30 g
Proteins: 3 g
Fats: 2 g

14. Almond Butter Toast with Blueberries

Preparation Time: 5 minutes
Portion Size: 2

Ingredients:

2 slices whole grain bread
2 tbsp almond butter
1/2 cup fresh blueberries

Instructions:

Toast bread slices.
Spread almond butter on each toast.
Top with fresh blueberries.
Serve immediately.

Nutrition Facts (1 portion):

Energy: 233 Kcal
Carbs: 29 g
Proteins: 8 g
Fats: 11 g

15. Chia Berry Yogurt Parfait

Preparation Time: 5 minutes
Resting Time: 2 hours
Portion Size: 2

Ingredients:

1 cup unsweetened almond milk
1/4 cup chia seeds
1 cup mixed berries
1 cup low-fat Greek yogurt
2 tbsp honey

Instructions:

Combine almond milk and chia seeds in a bowl, stir well and refrigerate for at least 2 hours.
In a glass, layer the chia pudding, mixed berries, and Greek yogurt.
Drizzle with honey.
Serve immediately or refrigerate until serving.

Nutrition Facts (1 portion):

Energy: 259 Kcal
Carbs: 41 g
Proteins: 11 g
Fats: 8 g

16. Veggie Omelet

Preparation Time: 10 minutes

Cooking Time: 5 minutes
Portion Size: 2

Ingredients:
4 large eggs
1 bell pepper, chopped
1 small onion, chopped
1 medium tomato, chopped
1 tbsp olive oil
Salt and pepper to taste

Instructions:
In a bowl, whisk the eggs, add salt and pepper, and set aside.
Heat the oil in a non-stick skillet, then add the bell pepper and onion. Sauté until they begin to soften.
Add the tomatoes and cook for another minute.
Pour the eggs over the vegetables and cook until set.
Fold the omelet in half and serve.

Nutrition Facts (1 portion):
Energy: 248 Kcal
Carbs: 11 g
Proteins: 14 g
Fats: 17 g

17. Avocado Tuna Salad
Preparation Time: 15 minutes
Portion Size: 2

Ingredients:
1 ripe avocado
1 can of tuna in water, drained
1/4 red onion, finely chopped
1 celery stalk, finely chopped
1 tablespoon of lemon juice
Salt and pepper to taste

Instructions:
In a bowl, mash the avocado with a fork until it's creamy.
Add the drained tuna, chopped onion, and chopped celery to the bowl.
Add the lemon juice, salt, and pepper, then mix well until all ingredients are combined.
Taste and adjust seasoning if needed.
Serve it on whole grain bread, lettuce leaves, or eat it as is!

Nutrition Facts (1 portion):
Energy: 270 Kcal
Carbs: 10 g
Proteins: 22 g
Fats: 17 g

18. Overnight Apple Cinnamon Oats
Preparation Time: 5 minutes
Resting Time: 8 hours
Portion Size: 2

Ingredients:
1 cup rolled oats
1 cup unsweetened almond milk
1 apple, chopped
1/2 tsp cinnamon
1 tbsp honey

Instructions:
Combine oats, almond milk, chopped apple, cinnamon, and honey in a jar.
Mix well, cover, and refrigerate overnight.
In the morning, give it a good stir and serve.

Nutrition Facts (1 portion):
Energy: 254 Kcal
Carbs: 52 g
Proteins: 6 g

Fats: 5 g

19. Blueberry Almond Milk Smoothie

Preparation Time: 5 minutes
Portion Size: 2

Ingredients:

1 banana
1 cup blueberries
1 cup unsweetened almond milk
1 tbsp chia seeds

Instructions:

Blend banana, blueberries, almond milk, and chia seeds in a blender until smooth.
Pour into glasses and serve immediately.

Nutrition Facts (1 portion):

Energy: 185 Kcal
Carbs: 40 g
Proteins: 4 g
Fats: 4 g

20. Tofu Scramble with Veggies

Preparation Time: 10 minutes
Cooking Time: 10 minutes
Portion Size: 2

Ingredients:

1 cup firm tofu, crumbled
1 bell pepper, chopped
1 small onion, chopped
1 medium tomato, chopped
1 tbsp olive oil
Salt and pepper to taste

Instructions:

Heat the oil in a skillet and sauté the bell pepper and onion until softened.
Add the crumbled tofu, tomato, salt, and pepper, and cook until heated through.
Serve hot.

Nutrition Facts (1 portion):

Energy: 243 Kcal
Carbs: 15 g
Proteins: 12 g
Fats: 16 g

Lunch

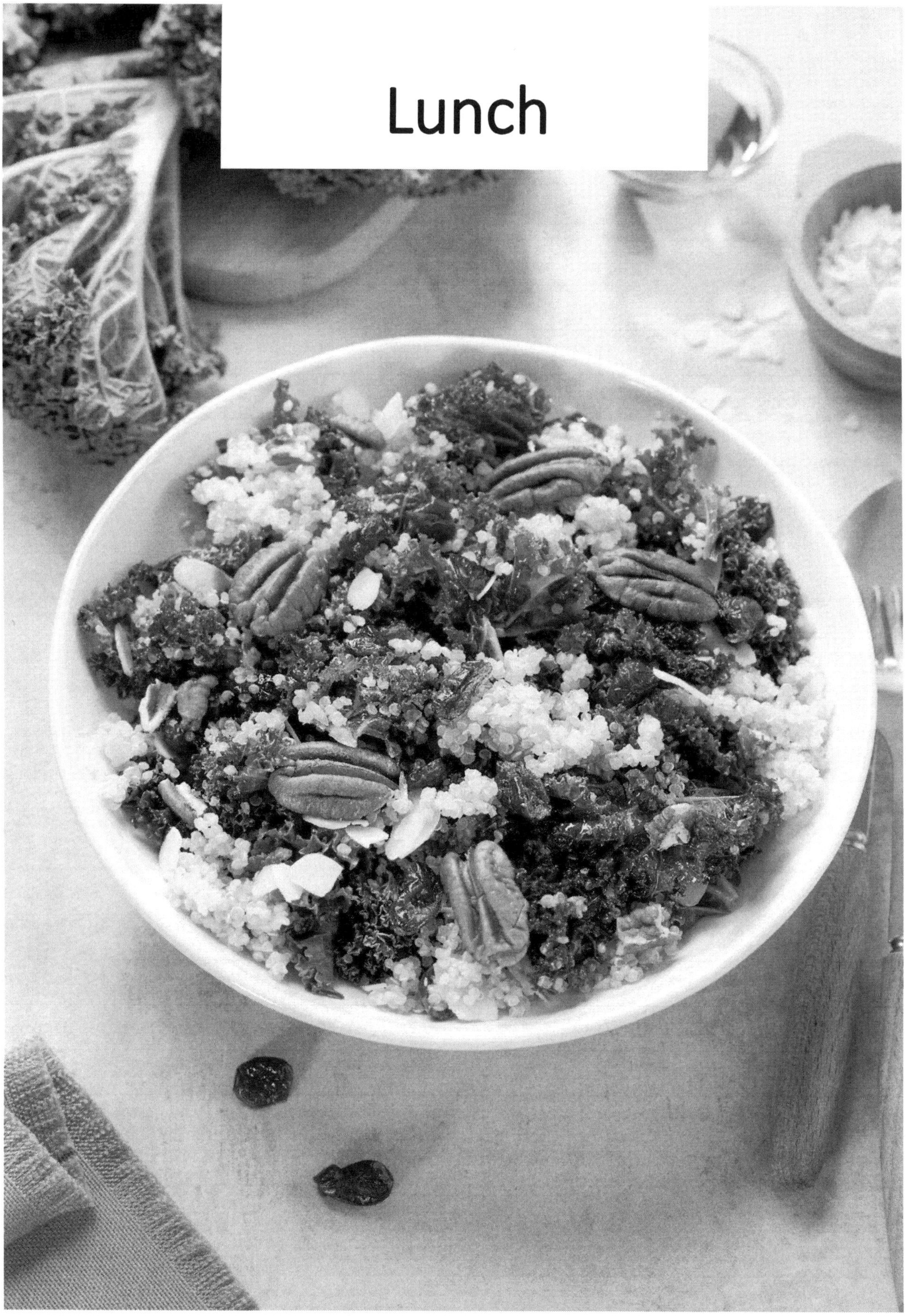

21. Quinoa Salad with Fresh Veggies

Preparation Time: 10 minutes
Cooking Time: 15 minutes
Portion Size: 2

Ingredients:

1/2 cup quinoa
1 cup water
1 cup diced cucumber
1/2 cup cherry tomatoes, halved
1/4 cup diced red onion
2 tbsp olive oil
1 tbsp lemon juice
Salt and pepper to taste

Instructions*:*

Cook the quinoa according to package ***instructions***.
Once cooked, let it cool and then transfer to a large bowl.
Add the cucumber, tomatoes, and red onion.
In a small bowl, whisk together the olive oil, lemon juice, salt, and pepper.
Pour the dressing over the salad and mix well.
Serve immediately or refrigerate for later.

Nutrition Facts (1 portion):

Energy: 295 Kcal
Carbs: 34 g
Proteins: 8 g
Fats: 15 g

22. Balsamic Grilled Chicken and Veggies

Preparation Time: 10 minutes
Cooking Time: 15 minutes
Portion Size: 2

Ingredients:

2 chicken breasts
1 zucchini, sliced
1 bell pepper, sliced
2 tbsp olive oil
2 tbsp balsamic vinegar
Salt and pepper to taste

Instructions:

Preheat your grill to medium heat.
Season the chicken and veggies with olive oil, balsamic vinegar, salt, and pepper.
Grill the chicken for 6-7 minutes on each side, and the veggies until they are tender.
Serve immediately.

Nutrition Facts (1 portion):

Energy: 335 Kcal
Carbs: 11 g
Proteins: 30 g
Fats: 18 g

23. Chickpea and Tomato Salad

Preparation Time: 10 minutes
Cooking Time: 0 minutes
Portion Size: 2

Ingredients:

1 can of chickpeas, drained and rinsed
2 large tomatoes, chopped
1 small red onion, finely chopped
1/4 cup fresh parsley, chopped
2 tablespoons olive oil
1 tablespoon lemon juice
Salt and pepper to taste

Instructions:

In a large bowl, combine the chickpeas, tomatoes, red onion, and parsley.
In a small bowl, whisk together the olive oil, lemon juice, salt, and pepper.

Pour the dressing over the salad and toss well to combine.
Let the salad sit for a few minutes to allow the flavors to meld together before serving.

Nutrition Facts (1 portion):
Energy: 280 Kcal
Carbs: 38 g
Proteins: 12 g
Fats: 11 g

24. Avocado and Black Bean Tacos

Preparation Time: 10 minutes
Cooking Time: 10 minutes
Portion Size: 2

Ingredients:
4 small whole grain tortillas
1 can black beans, drained and rinsed
1 avocado, sliced
1/2 cup salsa
1/2 cup shredded lettuce

Instructions:
Heat the black beans in a small saucepan over medium heat until warm.
Assemble the tacos by layering the beans, avocado slices, salsa, and lettuce on the tortillas.
Serve immediately.

Nutrition Facts (1 portion):
Energy: 380 Kcal
Carbs: 55 g
Proteins: 14 g
Fats: 13 g

25. Veggie-Packed Lentil Soup

Preparation Time: 10 minutes
Cooking Time: 30 minutes
Portion Size: 2

Ingredients:
1/2 cup green lentils
2 cups vegetable broth
1 carrot, diced
1 celery stalk, diced
1/2 onion, diced
2 garlic cloves, minced
1 tbsp olive oil
Salt and pepper to taste

Instructions:
In a pot, heat the olive oil over medium heat.
Add the onion, garlic, carrot, and celery and sauté until soft.
Add the lentils and broth. Bring to a boil, then reduce heat and simmer for about 30 minutes, or until lentils are tender.
Season with salt and pepper.
Serve hot.

Nutrition Facts (1 portion):
Energy: 275 Kcal
Carbs: 39 g
Proteins: 13 g
Fats: 7 g

26. Sweet Potato and Spinach Curry

Preparation Time: 15 minutes
Cooking Time: 30 minutes
Portion Size: 2

Ingredients:
2 sweet potatoes, peeled and cubed
2 cups fresh spinach
1 onion, diced
2 cloves garlic, minced
1 tbsp olive oil

1 tbsp curry powder
1 can coconut milk
Salt to taste

Instructions:

Heat olive oil in a pot over medium heat. Add onions and garlic, sauté until soft.
Add sweet potatoes and curry powder, stir to coat.
Pour in coconut milk, cover, and simmer until sweet potatoes are tender, about 20 minutes.
Add spinach and cook until wilted.
Season with salt to taste. Serve warm.

Nutrition Facts (1 portion):

Energy: 465 Kcal
Carbs: 58 g
Proteins: 9 g
Fats: 23 g

27. Turkey and Veggie Stir Fry

Preparation Time: 10 minutes
Cooking Time: 20 minutes
Portion Size: 2

Ingredients:

1/2 lb ground turkey
1 bell pepper, sliced
1 zucchini, sliced
1 onion, sliced
2 tbsp low sodium soy sauce
1 tbsp olive oil

Instructions:

Heat oil in a pan over medium heat. Add turkey and cook until browned.
Add vegetables and soy sauce, stir fry until vegetables are tender.
Serve hot.

Nutrition Facts (1 portion):

Energy: 285 Kcal
Carbs: 12 g
Proteins: 25 g
Fats: 15 g

28. Avocado Chicken Salad

Preparation Time: 15 minutes
Cooking Time: 0 minutes
Portion Size: 2

Ingredients:

2 cooked chicken breasts, shredded
1 ripe avocado, mashed
1/2 red onion, diced
1/2 cup chopped cilantro
Juice of 1 lime
Salt to taste

Instructions:

Combine all ingredients in a bowl, mix well.
Serve on whole grain bread or lettuce leaves.

Nutrition Facts (1 portion):

Energy: 340 Kcal
Carbs: 8 g
Proteins: 34 g
Fats: 18 g

29. Shrimp and Broccoli Stir Fry

Preparation Time: 10 minutes
Cooking Time: 10 minutes
Portion Size: 2

Ingredients:

1/2 lb shrimp, peeled and deveined
2 cups broccoli florets
2 cloves garlic, minced

2 tbsp low sodium soy sauce
1 tbsp olive oil

Instructions:

Heat oil in a pan over medium heat. Add garlic and shrimp, cook until shrimp is pink.
Add broccoli and soy sauce, stir fry until broccoli is tender.
Serve hot.

Nutrition Facts (1 portion):

Energy: 225 Kcal
Carbs: 10 g
Proteins: 25 g
Fats: 9 g

30. Veggie and Quinoa Stuffed Bell Peppers

Preparation Time: 15 minutes
Cooking Time: 30 minutes
Portion Size: 2

Ingredients:

2 bell peppers, tops removed and hollowed out
1/2 cup cooked quinoa
1/2 cup black beans, rinsed and drained
1/2 cup corn
1/2 cup shredded cheese
1/2 cup salsa

Instructions:

Preheat oven to 375°F. Place bell peppers in a baking dish.
Mix quinoa, beans, corn, cheese, and salsa in a bowl.
Stuff the mixture into the bell peppers.
Bake for 30 minutes or until the peppers are tender and the cheese is melted.
Serve hot.

Nutrition Facts (1 portion):

Energy: 340 Kcal
Carbs: 50 g
Proteins: 16 g
Fats: 10 g

31. Salmon with Lemon-Dill Sauce

Preparation Time: 10 minutes
Cooking Time: 15 minutes
Portion Size: 2

Ingredients:

2 salmon fillets
1 lemon, juiced
1 tbsp fresh dill, chopped
1 tbsp olive oil
Salt to taste

Instructions:

Preheat oven to 400°F. Place salmon on a baking sheet, drizzle with olive oil, and season with salt.
Bake for 12-15 minutes or until salmon is cooked through.
While the salmon is baking, combine lemon juice and dill in a small bowl to create the sauce.
Drizzle sauce over the cooked salmon before serving.

Nutrition Facts (1 portion):

Energy: 265 Kcal
Carbs: 2 g
Proteins: 34 g
Fats: 13 g

32. Butternut Squash Soup

Preparation Time: 10 minutes

Cooking Time: 40 minutes
Portion Size: 2

Ingredients:
1 small butternut squash, peeled and cubed
1 onion, diced
2 cloves garlic, minced
4 cups vegetable broth
1 tbsp olive oil
Salt to taste

Instructions:
Heat olive oil in a pot over medium heat. Add onions and garlic, sauté until soft.
Add butternut squash and broth, bring to a boil. Reduce heat and simmer until squash is tender, about 30 minutes.
Puree soup with a blender until smooth. Season with salt to taste. Serve warm.

Nutrition Facts (1 portion):
Energy: 210 Kcal
Carbs: 42 g
Proteins: 3 g
Fats: 5 g

33. Rainbow Salad Wraps

Preparation Time: 15 minutes
Cooking Time: 0 minutes
Portion Size: 2

Ingredients:
4 large lettuce leaves
1 carrot, shredded
1 beet, shredded
1/2 cucumber, sliced
1/2 bell pepper, sliced
1 avocado, sliced

Instructions:
Lay lettuce leaves flat. Evenly distribute carrot, beet, cucumber, bell pepper, and avocado among the leaves.
Roll up the lettuce leaves, tucking in the ends. Serve chilled.

Nutrition Facts (1 portion):
Energy: 180 Kcal
Carbs: 20 g
Proteins: 4 g
Fats: 11 g

34. Grilled Chicken and Veggie Skewers

Preparation Time: 15 minutes
Cooking Time: 15 minutes
Portion Size: 2

Ingredients:
1/2 lb chicken breast, cubed
1 bell pepper, cut into chunks
1 zucchini, cut into chunks
1 onion, cut into chunks
2 tbsp olive oil
Salt to taste

Instructions:
Preheat grill to medium heat. Thread chicken and vegetables onto skewers.
Brush skewers with olive oil and season with salt.
Grill skewers for 12-15 minutes or until chicken is cooked through, turning occasionally. Serve hot.

Nutrition Facts (1 portion):
Energy: 265 Kcal
Carbs: 12 g
Proteins: 28 g
Fats: 12 g

35. Mediterranean Quinoa Salad

Preparation Time: 15 minutes

Cooking Time: 15 minutes

Portion Size: 2

Ingredients:

1 cup cooked quinoa

1/2 cucumber, diced

1/2 bell pepper, diced

1/2 cup cherry tomatoes, halved

1/4 cup feta cheese, crumbled

1 tbsp olive oil

Juice of 1 lemon

Salt to taste

Instructions:

Combine all ingredients in a large bowl, mix well.

Serve chilled or at room temperature.

Nutrition Facts (1 portion):

Energy: 345 Kcal

Carbs: 45 g

Proteins: 12 g

Fats: 14 g

36. Lentil Stew

Preparation Time: 10 minutes

Cooking Time: 45 minutes

Portion Size: 2

Ingredients:

1 cup dry lentils

2 cups vegetable broth

1 onion, chopped

2 cloves garlic, minced

1 carrot, chopped

1 tsp olive oil

Salt to taste

Instructions:

Heat oil in a pot, add onions and garlic, sauté until soft.

Add lentils, broth, and carrots. Bring to a boil then reduce to a simmer, cook until lentils are tender, about 30-40 minutes.

Season with salt and serve warm.

Nutrition Facts (1 portion):

Energy: 315 Kcal

Carbs: 57 g

Proteins: 23 g

Fats: 2 g

37. Greek Lentil Salad

Preparation Time: 10 minutes

Portion Size: 2 servings

Ingredients:

1 cup cooked lentils

1 medium tomato, diced

1/2 cucumber, diced

1/2 red onion, thinly sliced

1/4 cup feta cheese, crumbled

1/4 cup olives, pitted and sliced

1 tablespoon olive oil

1 tablespoon red wine vinegar

Salt and pepper to taste

Instructions:

In a large bowl, combine cooked lentils, diced tomato, cucumber, red onion, feta cheese, and olives.

In a separate bowl, whisk together the olive oil, red wine vinegar, salt, and pepper to create the dressing.

Pour the dressing over the salad and toss until everything is well coated.

Let the salad sit for a few minutes to allow the flavors to blend together before serving.

Nutrition Facts (1 portion):

Energy: 340 Kcal

Carbs: 39 g

Proteins: 18 g

Fats: 14 g

38. Baked Sweet Potato

Preparation Time: 5 minutes

Cooking Time: 45 minutes

Portion Size: 2

Ingredients:

2 medium sweet potatoes

1 tbsp olive oil

Salt to taste

Instructions:

Preheat oven to 400°F. Coat sweet potatoes with olive oil and salt.

Place potatoes on a baking sheet and bake for 45 minutes or until soft.

Cut open and serve warm.

Nutrition Facts (1 portion):

Energy: 210 Kcal

Carbs: 45 g

Proteins: 4 g

Fats: 5 g

39. Avocado Chicken Salad

Preparation Time: 15 minutes

Portion Size: 2

Ingredients:

2 chicken breasts, cooked and shredded

1 ripe avocado

1 tablespoon of lemon juice

Salt and pepper to taste

4 cups of mixed salad greens

Instructions:

In a large bowl, mash the avocado until it's creamy.

Add the shredded chicken to the bowl and mix well until the chicken is coated with avocado.

Season with lemon juice, salt, and pepper. Mix well.

Serve the avocado chicken salad on a bed of mixed greens.

Enjoy it as a light lunch or dinner.

Nutrition Facts (1 portion):

Energy: 320 Kcal

Carbs: 8 g

Proteins: 38 g

Fats: 15 g

40. Turkey Lettuce Wraps

Preparation Time: 15 minutes

Cooking Time: 10 minutes

Portion Size: 2

Ingredients:

1/2 lb ground turkey

4 large lettuce leaves

1/2 onion, chopped

1 clove garlic, minced

1 tbsp olive oil

Salt to taste

Instructions:

Heat oil in a pan over medium heat. Add onion and garlic, sauté until soft.

Add turkey and cook until no longer pink. Season with salt.

Spoon turkey mixture onto lettuce leaves, roll up and serve.

Nutrition Facts (1 portion):

Energy: 270 Kcal

Carbs: 8 g

Proteins: 27 g

Fats: 15 g

Dinner

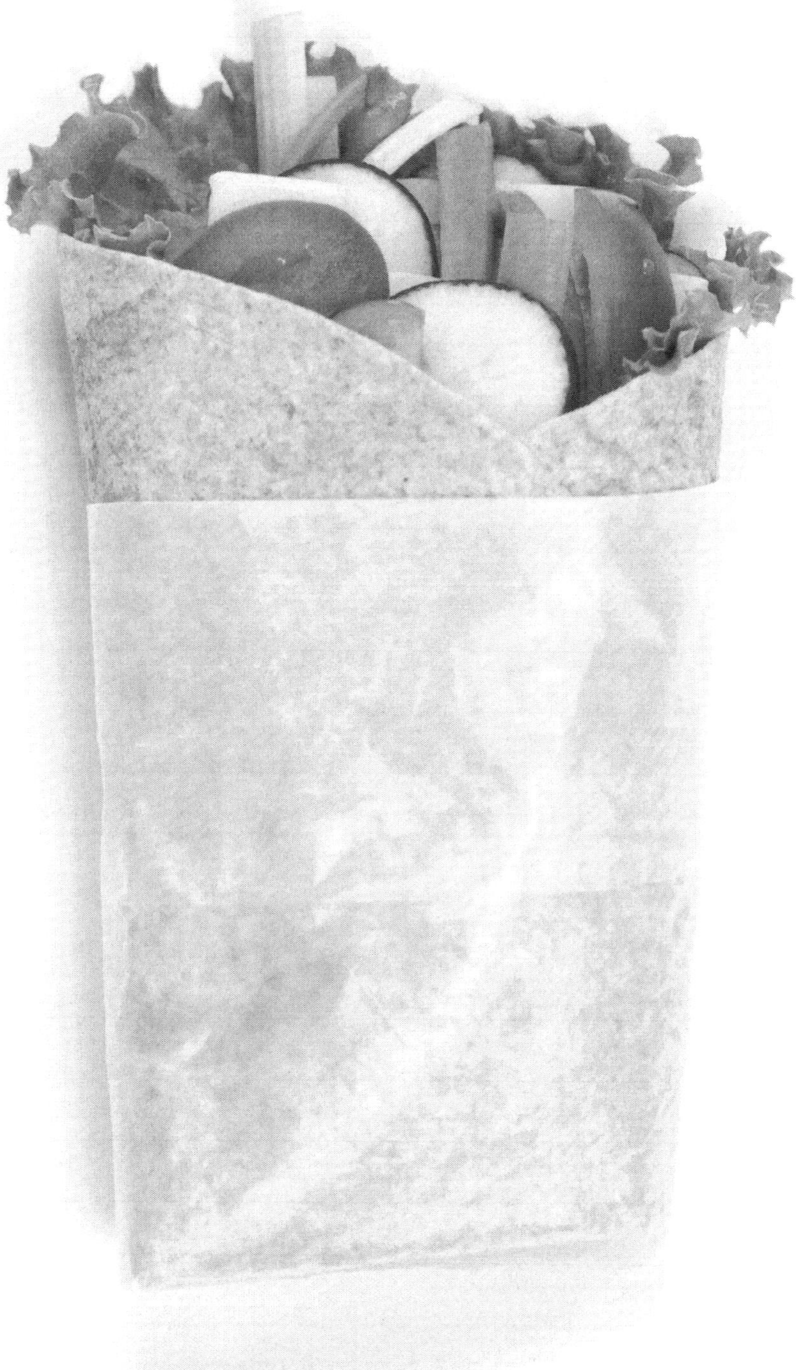

41. Greek Salad Wrap

Preparation Time: 15 minutes
Cooking Time: 0 minutes
Portion Size: 2

Ingredients:

2 whole grain tortillas
1 cup lettuce, chopped
1/2 cup cucumber, diced
1/2 cup tomato, diced
1/4 cup feta cheese
2 tbsp Greek dressing

Instructions:

Combine lettuce, cucumber, tomato, and feta cheese in a bowl. Drizzle with Greek dressing and toss well.
Divide the salad among the tortillas and roll up tightly.
Serve immediately.

Nutrition Facts (1 portion):

Energy: 218 Kcal
Carbs: 24 g
Proteins: 9 g
Fats: 11 g

42. Chickpea and Spinach Pasta

Preparation Time: 10 minutes
Cooking Time: 20 minutes
Portion Size: 2 servings

Ingredients:

4 ounces of your favorite pasta
1 tablespoon olive oil
2 cloves garlic, minced
1/2 medium onion, diced
1 can (7.5 ounces) chickpeas, drained and rinsed
1 cup of fresh spinach, roughly chopped
1/2 cup of vegetable broth
1/2 teaspoon of dried oregano
1/2 teaspoon of dried basil
Salt and pepper to taste
Grated vegan Parmesan cheese for garnish, optional

Instructions:

Cook the pasta according to the package instructions, then drain and set aside.
Meanwhile, heat the olive oil in a large skillet over medium heat.
Add the garlic and onion, and sauté until the onion becomes translucent.
Add the chickpeas, spinach, vegetable broth, oregano, basil, salt, and pepper to the skillet. Stir well.
Continue cooking for about 5-7 minutes, until the spinach has wilted and the chickpeas are heated through.
Toss the cooked pasta in the skillet with the other ingredients until everything is well combined.
Serve the pasta in bowls with a sprinkle of vegan Parmesan cheese on top, if desired.

Nutrition Facts (1 serving):

Energy: 470 Kcal
Carbs: 78 g
Proteins: 20 g
Fats: 10 g

43. Spinach and Goat Cheese Omelette

Preparation Time: 10 minutes
Cooking Time: 10 minutes
Portion Size: 2

Ingredients:

4 large eggs
2 cups spinach
1/4 cup goat cheese
1 tbsp olive oil
Salt and pepper to taste

Instructions:

Whisk eggs in a bowl. Set aside.
Heat oil in a non-stick skillet over medium heat. Add spinach and cook until wilted.
Pour in the eggs, sprinkle with cheese, and season with salt and pepper.
Cook until set, flip, and cook for another minute.
Serve hot.

Nutrition Facts (1 portion):

Energy: 296 Kcal
Carbs: 2 g
Proteins: 20 g
Fats: 22 g

44. Quinoa and Black Bean Salad

Preparation Time: 10 minutes
Cooking Time: 20 minutes
Portion Size: 2

Ingredients:

1/2 cup quinoa
1 cup water
1/2 cup black beans, drained and rinsed
1/2 cup corn kernels
1/4 cup chopped cilantro
2 tbsp lime juice
1 tbsp olive oil
Salt to taste

Instructions:

Rinse quinoa under cold water. In a pot, combine quinoa and water, bring to boil, reduce heat, cover and simmer until quinoa is cooked.
In a large bowl, combine cooked quinoa, black beans, corn, cilantro, lime juice, olive oil, and salt.
Serve immediately.

Nutrition Facts (1 portion):

Energy: 320 Kcal
Carbs: 52 g
Proteins: 14 g
Fats: 8 g

45. Grilled Salmon with Asparagus

Preparation Time: 10 minutes
Cooking Time: 20 minutes
Portion Size: 2

Ingredients:

2 4-oz salmon fillets
1 bunch asparagus
1 tbsp olive oil
Salt and pepper to taste

Instructions:

Brush salmon and asparagus with oil, season with salt and pepper, and grill until salmon is cooked to your liking and asparagus is tender.
Serve hot.

Nutrition Facts (1 portion):

Energy: 335 Kcal
Carbs: 5 g
Proteins: 35 g
Fats: 20 g

46. Pineapple & Tofu Stir-fry

Preparation Time: 10 minutes

Cooking Time: 15 minutes

Portion Size: 2

Ingredients:

1/2 cup tofu, cubed

1/2 cup pineapple chunks

1 cup bell peppers, sliced

1 tbsp olive oil

2 tbsp soy sauce

Instructions:

Heat oil in a skillet over medium heat. Add tofu cubes and fry until golden.

Add bell peppers and pineapple chunks, stir and cook for about 5 minutes.

Drizzle with soy sauce and stir well to combine.

Serve hot.

Nutrition Facts (1 portion):

Energy: 233 Kcal

Carbs: 20 g

Proteins: 11 g

Fats: 13 g

47. Shrimp Avocado Salad

Preparation Time: 15 minutes

Cooking Time: 5 minutes

Portion Size: 2

Ingredients:

1/2 lb cooked shrimp

1 avocado, diced

1/2 cup cherry tomatoes, halved

1/4 cup red onion, thinly sliced

1 tbsp lemon juice

1 tbsp olive oil

Salt and pepper to taste

Instructions:

Combine shrimp, avocado, cherry tomatoes, and red onion in a bowl.

Whisk together lemon juice, olive oil, salt, and pepper in a small bowl, then pour over the salad and toss to combine.

Serve immediately.

Nutrition Facts (1 portion):

Energy: 314 Kcal

Carbs: 12 g

Proteins: 24 g

Fats: 20 g

48. Chicken & Broccoli Stir-fry

Preparation Time: 10 minutes

Cooking Time: 15 minutes

Portion Size: 2

Ingredients:

1/2 lb chicken breast, cubed

1 cup broccoli florets

1/2 cup bell peppers, sliced

1 tbsp olive oil

2 tbsp soy sauce

Instructions:

Heat oil in a skillet over medium heat. Add chicken cubes and cook until no longer pink.

Add broccoli florets and bell pepper slices, stir and cook for about 5 minutes.

Drizzle with soy sauce and stir well to combine.

Serve hot.

Nutrition Facts (1 portion):

Energy: 244 Kcal

Carbs: 7 g

Proteins: 31 g

Fats: 10 g

49. Mediterranean Bulgur Salad

Preparation Time: 20 minutes
Portion Size: 2 servings

Ingredients:

1 cup cooked bulgur
1/2 cup diced cucumber
1/2 cup diced tomato
1/4 cup diced red onion
1/4 cup chopped kalamata olives
1/4 cup crumbled feta cheese
1/4 cup chopped fresh parsley
2 tablespoons olive oil
1 tablespoon lemon juice
Salt and pepper to taste

Instructions:

In a large bowl, combine cooked bulgur, cucumber, tomato, red onion, olives, feta cheese, and parsley.
In a separate bowl, whisk together the olive oil, lemon juice, salt, and pepper to create the dressing.
Pour the dressing over the salad and mix until well combined.
Allow the salad to sit for a few minutes for the flavors to blend together before serving.

Nutrition Facts (1 portion):

Energy: 385 Kcal
Carbs: 50 g
Proteins: 10 g
Fats: 18 g

50. Garlic Shrimp with Zucchini Noodles

Preparation Time: 15 minutes
Cooking Time: 10 minutes
Portion Size: 2

Ingredients:

1/2 lb shrimp, peeled and deveined
2 medium zucchinis
2 cloves garlic, minced
1 tbsp olive oil
Salt and pepper to taste

Instructions:

Using a spiralizer or a vegetable peeler, turn zucchinis into noodles.
Heat oil in a skillet over medium heat, add garlic and shrimp and cook until shrimp are pink and cooked through.
Add zucchini noodles, season with salt and pepper, and toss to combine.
Serve immediately.

Nutrition Facts (1 portion):

Energy: 214 Kcal
Carbs: 8 g
Proteins: 25 g
Fats: 9 g

51. Cauliflower Rice & Vegetables

Preparation Time: 15 minutes
Cooking Time: 10 minutes
Portion Size: 2

Ingredients:

2 cups cauliflower rice
1/2 cup bell peppers, sliced
1/2 cup zucchini, diced
1 tbsp olive oil
Salt and pepper to taste

Instructions:

Heat oil in a pan. Add the cauliflower rice, peppers, and zucchini.

Cook for 10 minutes, stirring frequently until vegetables are tender.

Season with salt and pepper.

Serve hot.

Nutrition Facts (1 portion):

Energy: 132 Kcal

Carbs: 12 g

Proteins: 5 g

Fats: 8 g

52. Ginger-Sesame Salmon

Preparation Time: 10 minutes

Cooking Time: 20 minutes

Portion Size: 2

Ingredients:

2 salmon fillets

1 tbsp sesame oil

1 tbsp soy sauce

1 tbsp grated fresh ginger

1/2 tbsp honey

Instructions:

Preheat the oven to 400 F.

Mix together sesame oil, soy sauce, ginger, and honey in a bowl.

Place the salmon fillets on a baking sheet and brush with the ginger-sesame mixture.

Bake for 20 minutes or until the salmon flakes easily with a fork.

Serve hot.

Nutrition Facts (1 portion):

Energy: 355 Kcal

Carbs: 6 g

Proteins: 34 g

Fats: 22 g

53. Quinoa & Black Bean Tacos

Preparation Time: 10 minutes

Cooking Time: 15 minutes

Portion Size: 2

Ingredients:

1/2 cup quinoa

1 cup canned black beans, rinsed

4 small corn tortillas

1 avocado, sliced

1/2 cup salsa

Instructions:

Cook the quinoa according to the package

Heat the black beans in a small pot.

To assemble the tacos, spread a layer of quinoa on each tortilla, then top with black beans, avocado slices, and salsa.

Serve immediately.

Nutrition Facts (1 portion):

Energy: 428 Kcal

Carbs: 64 g

Proteins: 16 g

Fats: 15 g

54. Zucchini & Yellow Squash Soup

Preparation Time: 10 minutes

Cooking Time: 20 minutes

Portion Size: 2

Ingredients:

1 zucchini, diced

1 yellow squash, diced

1 onion, diced

1 tbsp olive oil

2 cups vegetable broth

Salt and pepper to taste

Instructions:

In a pot, heat the oil and add the onion, zucchini, and squash. Cook until tender.
Add the broth and bring to a boil. Reduce heat and simmer for 20 minutes.
Blend the soup until smooth.
Season with salt and pepper.
Serve hot.

Nutrition Facts (1 portion):

Energy: 131 Kcal
Carbs: 16 g
Proteins: 3 g
Fats: 7 g

55. Greek Yogurt Chicken

Preparation Time: 10 minutes
Cooking Time: 30 minutes
Portion Size: 2

Ingredients:

2 chicken breasts
1/2 cup Greek yogurt
1 tbsp lemon juice
1 tbsp dried oregano
1 clove garlic, minced
Salt and pepper to taste

Instructions:

Preheat the oven to 375 F.
In a bowl, combine Greek yogurt, lemon juice, oregano, garlic, salt, and pepper.
Coat the chicken breasts in the yogurt mixture.
Bake for 30 minutes or until chicken is cooked through.
Serve hot.

Nutrition Facts (1 portion):

Energy: 280 Kcal
Carbs: 5 g
Proteins: 55 g
Fats: 4 g

56. Spaghetti Squash with Cherry Tomatoes

Preparation Time: 15 minutes
Cooking Time: 40 minutes
Portion Size: 2

Ingredients:

1 spaghetti squash
1 cup cherry tomatoes, halved
1 tbsp olive oil
Salt and pepper to taste

Instructions:

Preheat oven to 375°F. Cut the squash in half lengthwise, scoop out seeds, and place cut-side down on a baking sheet.
Bake for about 40 minutes or until the flesh is tender. Once cool enough to handle, scrape out the spaghetti-like strands with a fork.
In a pan, heat oil and sauté the tomatoes until soft.
Toss the squash strands with the tomatoes, season with salt and pepper, and serve.

Nutrition Facts (1 portion):

Energy: 212 Kcal
Carbs: 32 g
Proteins: 3 g
Fats: 9 g

57. Lemon-Dill Grilled Shrimp

Preparation Time: 10 minutes

Cooking Time: 5 minutes
Portion Size: 2

Ingredients:

1 lb large shrimp, peeled and deveined
1 tbsp olive oil
Juice of 1 lemon
1 tsp dried dill
Salt and pepper to taste

Instructions:

Preheat grill to medium-high heat.
Toss shrimp in oil, lemon juice, dill, salt, and pepper.
Grill for about 2-3 minutes per side, until opaque.
Serve immediately.

Nutrition Facts (1 portion):

Energy: 242 Kcal
Carbs: 2 g
Proteins: 46 g
Fats: 5 g

58. Mediterranean Tofu Stir-Fry

Preparation Time: 10 minutes
Cooking Time: 10 minutes
Portion Size: 2

Ingredients:

1 block tofu, cubed
1 cup bell peppers, sliced
1/2 cup red onion, sliced
1 tbsp olive oil
Salt and pepper to taste

Instructions:

Heat oil in a pan, add tofu cubes and cook until golden brown.
Add the peppers and onion, sauté until tender.
Season with salt and pepper and serve.

Nutrition Facts (1 portion):

Energy: 338 Kcal
Carbs: 16 g
Proteins: 22 g
Fats: 22 g

59. Baked Cod with Lemon & Parsley

Preparation Time: 10 minutes
Cooking Time: 15 minutes
Portion Size: 2

Ingredients:

2 cod fillets
Juice of 1 lemon
1 tbsp olive oil
2 tbsp chopped fresh parsley
Salt and pepper to taste

Instructions:

Preheat oven to 400°F.
Place cod in a baking dish. Drizzle with lemon juice and oil, then sprinkle with parsley, salt, and pepper.
Bake for about 15 minutes, until fish flakes easily with a fork.
Serve immediately.

Nutrition Facts (1 portion):

Energy: 226 Kcal
Carbs: 2 g
Proteins: 40 g
Fats: 7 g

60. Quinoa Salad with Avocado & Cucumber

Preparation Time: 10 minutes
Cooking Time: 15 minutes

Portion Size: 2

Ingredients:

1/2 cup quinoa
1 cucumber, diced
1 avocado, diced
1 tbsp olive oil
Juice of 1 lemon
Salt and pepper to taste

Instructions:

Cook the quinoa according to the package
In a large bowl, combine the cooked quinoa, cucumber, and avocado.
Whisk together the oil, lemon juice, salt, and pepper, then drizzle over the salad.
Toss well and serve.

Nutrition Facts (1 portion):

Energy: 350 Kcal
Carbs: 39 g
Proteins: 8 g
Fats: 20 g

Side Dish

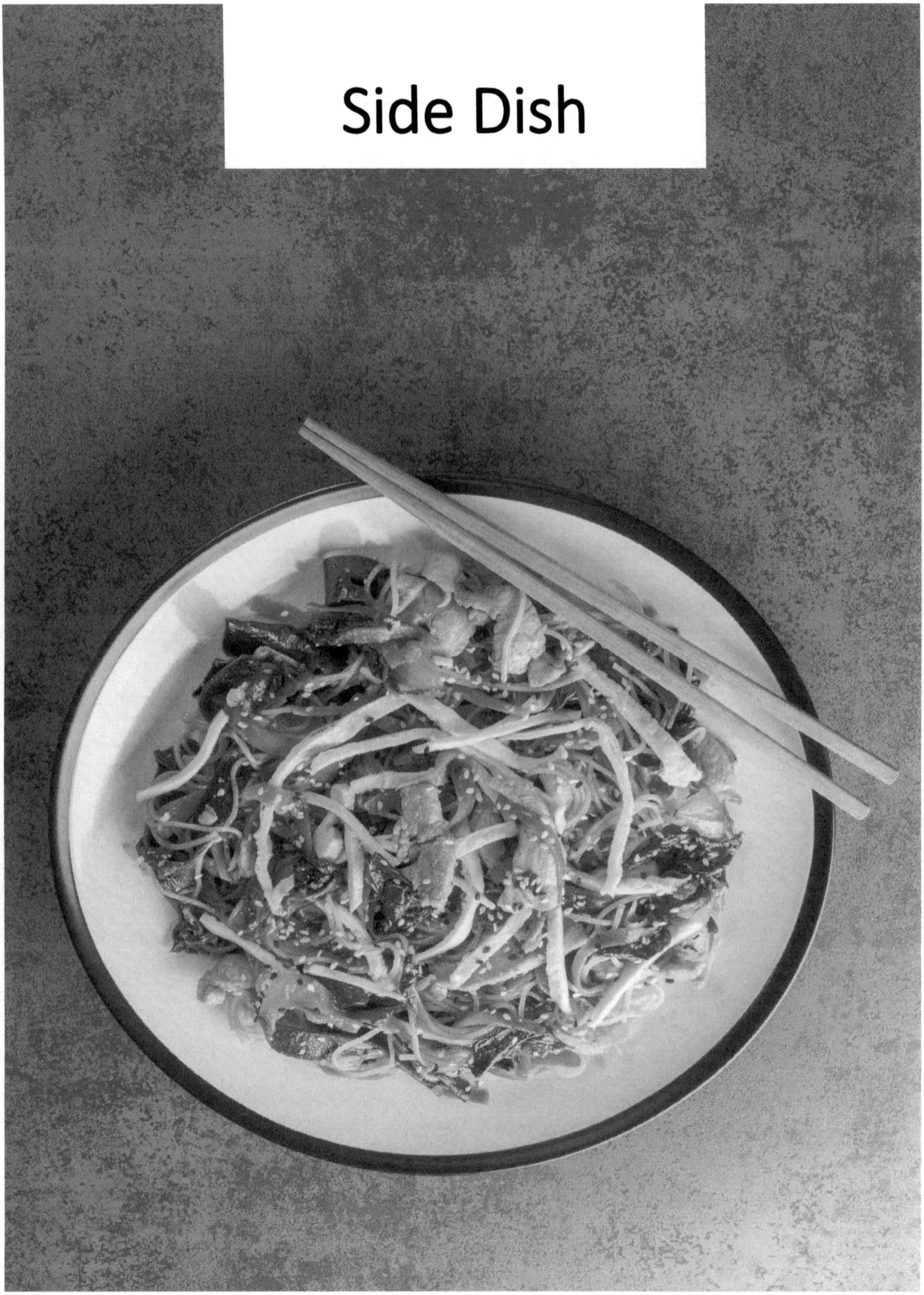

61. Apple Cider Vinegar Brussels Sprouts

Preparation Time: 10 minutes
Cooking Time: 25 minutes
Portion Size: 2

Ingredients:

1 lb Brussels sprouts, trimmed and halved
1 tbsp olive oil
2 tbsp apple cider vinegar
Salt and pepper to taste

Instructions:

Preheat the oven to 400°F.
Toss the Brussels sprouts in olive oil, apple cider vinegar, salt, and pepper.
Spread them on a baking sheet and roast for 25 minutes or until they are golden and crispy.

Nutrition Facts (1 portion):

Energy: 148 Kcal
Carbs: 19 g
Proteins: 7 g
Fats: 7 g

62. Spinach and Mushroom Stir-Fry

Preparation Time: 10 minutes
Cooking Time: 15 minutes
Portion Size: 2

Ingredients:

2 cups fresh spinach
1 cup sliced mushrooms
1 tbsp olive oil
2 cloves garlic, minced
Salt and pepper to taste

Instructions:

Heat the olive oil in a pan over medium heat.
Add the garlic and mushrooms. Cook for about 5 minutes, until the mushrooms are golden.
Add the spinach and stir until it wilts.
Season with salt and pepper to taste.

Nutrition Facts (1 portion):

Energy: 93 Kcal
Carbs: 5 g
Proteins: 3 g
Fats: 7 g

63. Lemon Dill Cucumber Salad

Preparation Time: 15 minutes
Cooking Time: 0 minutes
Portion Size: 2

Ingredients:

2 large cucumbers, thinly sliced
2 tbsp fresh dill, chopped
2 tbsp lemon juice
1 tbsp olive oil
Salt to taste

Instructions:

In a large bowl, combine cucumber slices, dill, lemon juice, and olive oil. Toss to combine.
Season with salt to taste. Let the salad sit for a few minutes to allow the flavors to meld.

Nutrition Facts (1 portion):

Energy: 80 Kcal
Carbs: 5 g
Proteins: 1 g
Fats: 7 g

64. Roasted Beet and Walnut Salad

Preparation Time: 10 minutes

Cooking Time: 45 minutes
Portion Size: 2

Ingredients:
2 medium beets
1/4 cup chopped walnuts
2 cups mixed greens
1 tbsp olive oil
Salt and pepper to taste

Instructions:
Preheat the oven to 400°F. Wrap the beets in foil and roast for 45 minutes or until tender. Once cool, peel and chop the beets.
Toss the beets, walnuts, and mixed greens in olive oil. Season with salt and pepper.

Nutrition Facts (1 portion):
Energy: 205 Kcal
Carbs: 13 g
Proteins: 4 g
Fats: 16 g

65. Garlic Roasted Broccoli
Preparation Time: 10 minutes
Cooking Time: 20 minutes
Portion Size: 2

Ingredients:
2 cups broccoli florets
2 cloves garlic, minced
1 tbsp olive oil
Salt and pepper to taste

Instructions:
Preheat your oven to 400°F.
In a bowl, mix the broccoli florets with garlic, olive oil, salt, and pepper.
Arrange the broccoli on a baking sheet in a single layer.
Roast for 20 minutes or until the broccoli is crispy and golden.

Nutrition Facts (1 portion):
Energy: 111 Kcal
Carbs: 8 g
Proteins: 4 g
Fats: 8 g

66. Ginger Turmeric Carrots
Preparation Time: 10 minutes
Cooking Time: 15 minutes
Portion Size: 2

Ingredients:
5 medium carrots, sliced
1 tbsp olive oil
1 tsp grated ginger
1 tsp grated turmeric
Salt to taste

Instructions:
Heat the olive oil in a pan over medium heat. Add the carrots, ginger, and turmeric. Cook for about 15 minutes, until the carrots are tender.
Season with salt to taste.

Nutrition Facts (1 portion):
Energy: 134 Kcal
Carbs: 20 g
Proteins: 2 g
Fats: 7 g

67. Quinoa & Green Beans Salad
Preparation Time: 10 minutes
Cooking Time: 20 minutes
Portion Size: 2

Ingredients:
1 cup cooked quinoa
1 cup fresh green beans, cut into 1-inch pieces
1 tbsp olive oil
1 tbsp lemon juice
Salt and pepper to taste

Instructions:
In a pot of boiling water, cook the green beans for about 5 minutes. Drain and set aside.
In a bowl, mix the quinoa, green beans, olive oil, and lemon juice.
Season with salt and pepper.

Nutrition Facts (1 portion):
Energy: 237 Kcal
Carbs: 35 g
Proteins: 8 g
Fats: 9 g

68. Garlic & Lemon Zucchini Noodles
Preparation Time: 10 minutes
Cooking Time: 10 minutes
Portion Size: 2

Ingredients:
2 medium zucchinis, spiraled into noodles
2 cloves garlic, minced
1 tbsp olive oil
1 tbsp lemon juice
Salt and pepper to taste

Instructions:
In a pan over medium heat, sauté the garlic in olive oil for about 2 minutes.
Add the zucchini noodles and cook for another 2 minutes.
Stir in the lemon juice and season with salt and pepper.

Nutrition Facts (1 portion):
Energy: 105 Kcal
Carbs: 8 g
Proteins: 3 g
Fats: 8 g

69. Mashed Sweet Potatoes
Preparation Time: 5 minutes
Cooking Time: 20 minutes
Portion Size: 2

Ingredients:
2 medium sweet potatoes, peeled and cubed
1 tbsp olive oil
Salt and pepper to taste

Instructions:
Boil the sweet potatoes until tender, about 20 minutes. Drain.
Mash the potatoes with olive oil, salt, and pepper until smooth.

Nutrition Facts (1 portion):
Energy: 175 Kcal
Carbs: 31 g
Proteins: 2 g
Fats: 7 g

70. Avocado & Tomato Salad
Preparation Time: 10 minutes
Cooking Time: 0 minutes
Portion Size: 2

Ingredients:
1 large avocado, diced
2 medium tomatoes, diced

1 tbsp lemon juice
1 tbsp olive oil
Salt and pepper to taste

Instructions:
In a bowl, combine avocado, tomatoes, lemon juice, and olive oil. Gently toss.
Season with salt and pepper.

Nutrition Facts (1 portion):
Energy: 235 Kcal
Carbs: 12 g
Proteins: 3 g
Fats: 21 g

71. Greek-Style Cucumbers

Preparation Time: 10 minutes
Cooking Time: 0 minutes
Portion Size: 2

Ingredients:
2 cucumbers, sliced
1/4 cup feta cheese, crumbled
2 tbsp olive oil
1 tbsp lemon juice
Salt and pepper to taste

Instructions:
Combine all ingredients in a bowl and gently toss.
Serve immediately.

Nutrition Facts (1 portion):
Energy: 195 Kcal
Carbs: 6 g
Proteins: 5 g
Fats: 18 g

72. Sautéed Brussels Sprouts

Preparation Time: 5 minutes
Cooking Time: 10 minutes
Portion Size: 2

Ingredients:
2 cups Brussels sprouts, halved
1 tbsp olive oil
Salt and pepper to taste
Instructions*:*
Heat the olive oil in a pan over medium heat.
Add the Brussels sprouts and cook until they start to brown, about 10 minutes.
Season with salt and pepper.

Nutrition Facts (1 portion):
Energy: 107 Kcal
Carbs: 10 g
Proteins: 4 g
Fats: 7 g

73. Sweet Potato & Beet Salad

Preparation Time: 15 minutes
Cooking Time: 30 minutes
Portion Size: 2

Ingredients:
1 large sweet potato, peeled and cubed
2 small beets, peeled and cubed
1 tbsp olive oil
Salt and pepper to taste

Instructions:
Roast the sweet potatoes and beets in a preheated oven at 400°F for 30 minutes.
Toss with olive oil, salt, and pepper.

Nutrition Facts (1 portion):
Energy: 212 Kcal
Carbs: 31 g
Proteins: 4 g
Fats: 9 g

74. Garlic Asparagus

Preparation Time: 10 minutes
Cooking Time: 15 minutes
Portion Size: 2 servings

Ingredients:

1 bunch of asparagus (about 1/2 lb or 225 g)
2 cloves of garlic, minced
1 tablespoon of olive oil
Salt and black pepper to taste
Lemon wedges (optional)

Instructions:

Trim the bottom ends of the asparagus spears, as they can be tough and woody.
Heat the olive oil in a large frying pan over medium heat. Sauté the minced garlic for a minute, or until it becomes aromatic. Make sure not to burn the garlic.
Toss in the asparagus spears. Cook, stirring periodically, for approximately 10 minutes, or until the asparagus is tender and slightly crunchy. If the asparagus is quite thick, cover the pan to allow it to steam for a few minutes.
Season to taste with salt and pepper. Serve with lemon wedges for a punch of freshness if preferred.

Nutrition Facts (1 serving):

Energy: 90 Kcal
Carbs: 6 g
Proteins: 3 g
Fats: 7 g

75. Turmeric Roasted Cauliflower

Preparation Time: 10 minutes
Cooking Time: 30 minutes
Portion Size: 2

Ingredients:

1/2 head of cauliflower, cut into florets
1 tbsp olive oil
1 tsp turmeric
Salt and pepper to taste

Instructions:

Preheat oven to 400°F.
Toss cauliflower with olive oil, turmeric, salt, and pepper.
Roast for 30 minutes until golden and crispy.

Nutrition Facts (1 portion):

Energy: 106 Kcal
Carbs: 8 g
Proteins: 3 g
Fats: 8 g

76. Grilled Zucchini

Preparation Time: 10 minutes
Cooking Time: 15 minutes
Portion Size: 2

Ingredients:

2 medium zucchinis, sliced
1 tbsp olive oil
Salt and pepper to taste

Instructions*:*

Brush zucchini slices with olive oil, season with salt and pepper.
Grill until tender and slightly charred.

Nutrition Facts (1 portion):

Energy: 107 Kcal
Carbs: 5 g
Proteins: 2 g
Fats: 9 g

77. Quinoa & Tempeh Stir Fry

Preparation Time: 15 minutes

Cooking Time: 15 minutes

Portion Size: 2 servings

Ingredients:

1 cup cooked quinoa

100 grams tempeh, cut into small cubes

2 cups mixed vegetables (like bell peppers, broccoli, carrots), chopped

2 cloves garlic, minced

2 tablespoons soy sauce (or tamari for gluten-free option)

1 tablespoon sesame oil (or any cooking oil)

1 teaspoon grated fresh ginger

Optional toppings: sesame seeds, chopped green onions

Instructions:

Heat the oil in a large pan or wok over medium heat. Add the tempeh cubes and cook until they are browned on all sides. Remove the tempeh from the pan and set aside.

In the same pan, add more oil if necessary, then add the garlic and ginger. Cook for about a minute until fragrant.

Stir in the chopped veggies for approximately 5-7 minutes, or until they are tender-crisp.

Return the cooked quinoa and fried tempeh to the pan. To incorporate with the veggies, stir well.

Pour the soy sauce over the mixture and whisk well. Cook for another 2-3 minutes, or until everything is well heated.

Serve the stir fry in bowls, if preferred garnished with sesame seeds and sliced green onions.

Nutrition Facts (1 serving):

Energy: 350 Kcal

Carbs: 46 g

Proteins: 18 g

Fats: 11 g

78. Cucumber Tomato Salad

Preparation Time: 10 minutes

Cooking Time: 0 minutes

Portion Size: 2

Ingredients:

2 medium cucumbers, chopped

2 medium tomatoes, chopped

1/4 cup red onion, thinly sliced

2 tbsp olive oil

1 tbsp apple cider vinegar

Salt and pepper to taste

Instructions:

In a bowl, combine cucumbers, tomatoes, and onion.

Drizzle with olive oil and vinegar, season with salt and pepper. Toss to combine.

Nutrition Facts (1 portion):

Energy: 161 Kcal

Carbs: 11 g

Proteins: 2 g

Fats: 14 g

79. Sautéed Spinach with Garlic

Preparation Time: 5 minutes

Cooking Time: 5 minutes

Portion Size: 2

Ingredients:

4 cups fresh spinach

2 garlic cloves, minced

1 tbsp olive oil

Salt and pepper to taste

Instructions:

Heat oil in a pan, add garlic and cook until fragrant.

Add spinach and sauté until wilted. Season with salt and pepper.

Nutrition Facts (1 portion):

Energy: 94 Kcal

Carbs: 3 g

Proteins: 2 g

Fats: 8 g

80. Roasted Sweet Potato Wedges

Preparation Time: 10 minutes

Cooking Time: 30 minutes

Portion Size: 2

Ingredients:

2 medium sweet potatoes, cut into wedges

1 tbsp olive oil

Salt and pepper to taste

Instructions:

Preheat oven to 400°F.

Toss sweet potato wedges with olive oil, salt, and pepper.

Roast for 30 minutes until tender and slightly crispy.

Nutrition Facts (1 portion):

Energy: 206 Kcal

Carbs: 29 g

Proteins: 2 g

Fats: 10 g

Vegan and Vegetarian

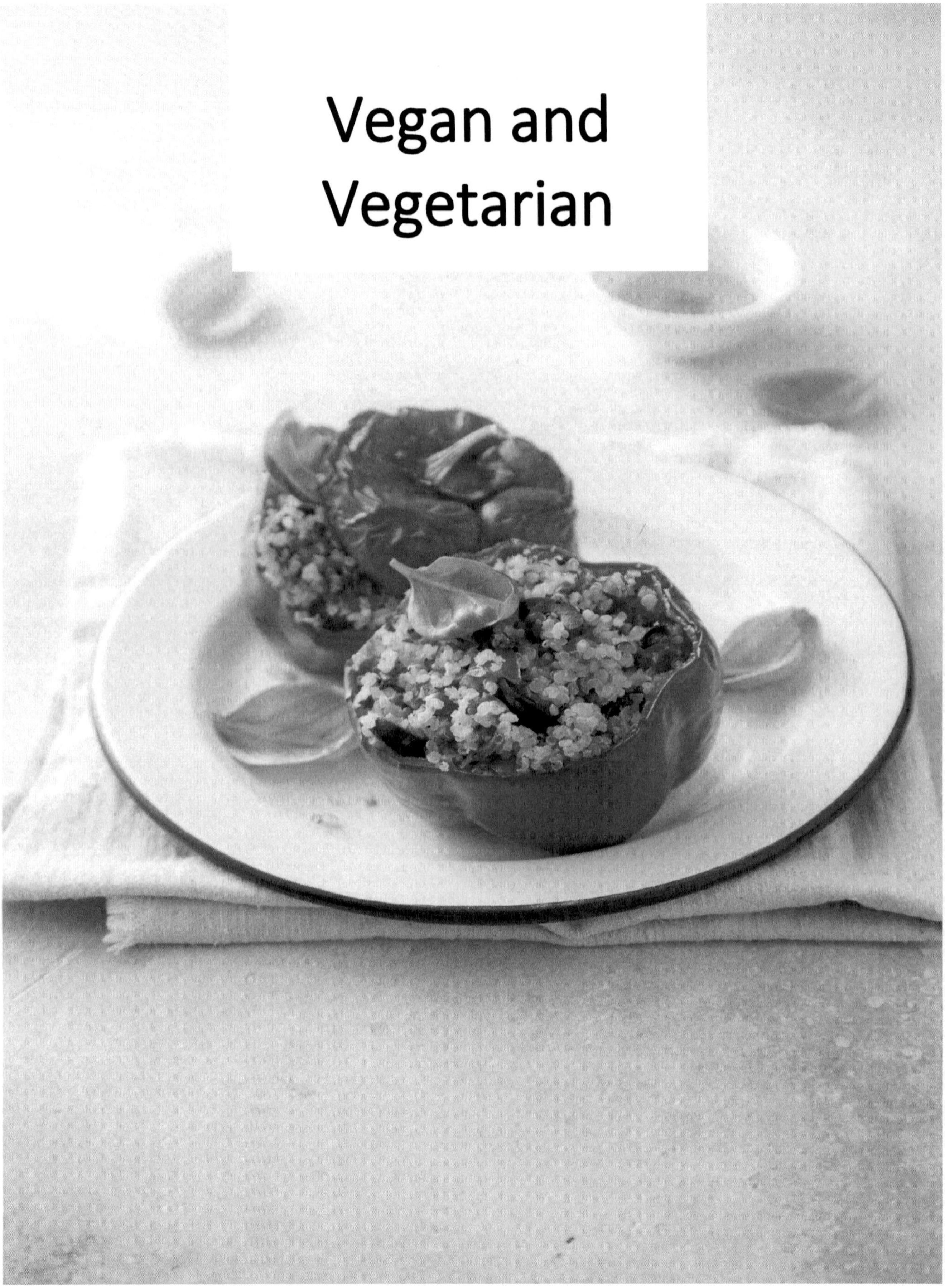

81. Vegan Quinoa Stuffed Bell Peppers

Preparation Time: 15 minutes
Cooking Time: 30 minutes
Portion Size: 2

Ingredients:

2 large bell peppers, any color
1/2 cup cooked quinoa
1/2 cup black beans, rinsed and drained
1/2 cup corn kernels, fresh or frozen
1/4 cup diced tomatoes
1 tbsp olive oil
Salt and pepper to taste

Instructions:

Preheat oven to 375°F.
Remove the tops and seeds from the bell peppers.
In a mixing dish, combine the cooked quinoa, black beans, corn, and diced tomatoes.
Season with salt and pepper to taste.
Stuff the quinoa mixture inside the bell peppers.
Place the peppers in a baking dish, sprinkle with olive oil, and bake for 30 minutes, or until soft..
Serve hot.

Nutrition Facts (1 portion):

Energy: 288 Kcal
Carbs: 49 g
Proteins: 11 g
Fats: 8 g

82. Vegan Peanut Butter Banana Smoothie

Preparation Time: 5 minutes
Cooking Time: 0 minutes
Portion Size: 2

Ingredients:

2 bananas
2 cups almond milk
2 tbsp natural peanut butter
1 tsp chia seeds

Instructions:

Combine bananas, almond milk, and peanut butter in a blender.
Blend until smooth.
Pour into glasses and top with chia seeds.
Serve immediately.

Nutrition Facts (1 portion):

Energy: 308 Kcal
Carbs: 42 g
Proteins: 8 g
Fats: 15 g

83. Vegan Berry Chia Pudding

Preparation Time: 10 minutes
Cooking Time: 0 minutes (plus refrigeration time)
Portion Size: 2

Ingredients:

1/4 cup chia seeds
1 cup almond milk
1 tbsp maple syrup
1/2 cup mixed berries

Instructions:

In a bowl, combine chia seeds, almond milk, and maple syrup.
Stir well, cover, and refrigerate for at least 2 hours or overnight.

Once the pudding is set, top with mixed berries before serving.
Serve chilled.

Nutrition Facts (1 portion):
Energy: 195 Kcal
Carbs: 28 g
Proteins: 5 g
Fats: 8 g

84. Vegan Balsamic Grilled Vegetables

Preparation Time: 10 minutes
Cooking Time: 15 minutes
Portion Size: 2

Ingredients:
1 zucchini, sliced lengthwise
1 bell pepper, sliced
1/2 eggplant, sliced
2 tbsp olive oil
1 tbsp balsamic vinegar
Salt and pepper to taste

Instructions:
Preheat grill to medium heat.
Toss vegetables with olive oil, balsamic vinegar, salt, and pepper.
Grill vegetables for about 5-7 minutes on each side, until tender and charred.
Serve hot.

Nutrition Facts (1 portion):
Energy: 183 Kcal
Carbs: 15 g
Proteins: 3 g
Fats: 14 g

85. Vegan Stuffed Avocados

Preparation Time: 10 minutes
Cooking Time: 0 minutes
Portion Size: 2

Ingredients:
1 large ripe avocado, halved and pitted
1/2 cup chickpeas, rinsed and drained
1/4 cup diced tomato
1/4 cup diced cucumber
1 tbsp olive oil
1/2 lemon, juiced
Salt and pepper to taste

Instructions:
In a bowl, mix together chickpeas, tomato, cucumber, olive oil, and lemon juice. Season with salt and pepper.
Scoop the mixture into the avocado halves.
Serve immediately.

Nutrition Facts (1 portion):
Energy: 329 Kcal
Carbs: 21 g
Proteins: 6 g
Fats: 27 g

86. Vegan Sweet Potato and Black Bean Tacos

Preparation Time: 15 minutes
Cooking Time: 15 minutes
Portion Size: 2

Ingredients:
4 small corn tortillas
1 large sweet potato, diced
1/2 cup black beans, rinsed and drained
1/2 onion, diced
1 clove garlic, minced
1 tbsp olive oil
Salt and pepper to taste

Instructions:

Heat the olive oil in a pan over medium heat.
Add the onion and garlic, sauté until onion is translucent.
Add the sweet potato, cook until tender.
Stir in the black beans, season with salt and pepper.
Warm the tortillas in a dry skillet, then top with the sweet potato and black bean mixture.
Serve hot.

Nutrition Facts (1 portion):

Energy: 314 Kcal
Carbs: 53 g
Proteins: 9 g
Fats: 9 g

87. Vegan Veggie Stir-Fry with Tofu

Preparation Time: 10 minutes
Cooking Time: 15 minutes
Portion Size: 2

Ingredients:

4 oz firm tofu, cubed
1 bell pepper, sliced
1 zucchini, sliced
1 carrot, sliced
2 tbsp low-sodium soy sauce
1 tbsp olive oil

Instructions:

Heat the olive oil in a large pan or wok over medium heat.
Cook until the tofu is browned on both sides.
Stir-fry the bell pepper, zucchini, and carrot for approximately 5 minutes, or until the veggies are tender-crisp.
Stir in the soy sauce to cover the tofu and veggies.
Serve hot.

Nutrition Facts (1 portion):

Energy: 195 Kcal
Carbs: 15 g
Proteins: 9 g
Fats: 12 g

88. Vegan Split Pea Soup

Preparation Time: 1 hour 10 minutes
Portion Size: 2 servings

Ingredients:

1/2 cup dried split peas
1/2 large onion, diced
1 carrot, diced
1 celery stalk, diced
1 garlic clove, minced
1 1/2 cups vegetable broth
1/4 teaspoon dried thyme
1/4 teaspoon black pepper
Salt to taste

Instructions:

Rinse the split peas under cold water.
Sauté the onion, carrot, celery, and garlic in a tiny quantity of vegetable stock in a medium saucepan until the onion is translucent, approximately 5-7 minutes.
Add the split peas, the remaining vegetable broth, thyme, and black pepper to taste.
Bring the water to a boil.
Reduce the heat to low, cover the saucepan, and cook for 1 hour, or until the split peas are soft. Stir periodically and, if necessary, add additional water.
Puree the soup with an immersion blender until smooth. If you don't have an immersion

blender, you may puree the soup in a conventional blender before returning it to the pot. Take caution since the soup will be hot.

If necessary, season the soup with salt.

Serve immediately with crusty bread.

If you like a chunkier soup, omit the blending stage or mix just a part of the soup.

Nutrition Facts (1 serving):

Energy: 280 Kcal

Carbs: 50 g

Proteins: 20 g

Fats: 1.5 g

89. Vegan Tomato and Basil Bruschetta

Preparation Time: 10 minutes

Cooking Time: 5 minutes

Portion Size: 2

Ingredients:

4 slices whole grain bread

1 large tomato, diced

1/4 cup fresh basil leaves, chopped

1 clove garlic, minced

1 tbsp olive oil

Salt and pepper to taste

Instructions:

Toast the bread slices.

In a bowl, combine the diced tomato, chopped basil, minced garlic, olive oil, salt, and pepper.

Spoon the tomato mixture onto the toasted bread slices.

Serve immediately.

Nutrition Facts (1 portion):

Energy: 217 Kcal

Carbs: 27 g

Proteins: 7 g

Fats: 10 g

90. Vegan Almond Butter and Banana Toast

Preparation Time: 5 minutes

Cooking Time: 2 minutes

Portion Size: 2

Ingredients:

4 slices whole grain bread

2 tbsp almond butter

1 banana, sliced

Instructions:

Toast the bread slices.

Spread the almond butter onto the toasted bread slices.

Top with banana slices.

Serve immediately.

Nutrition Facts (1 portion):

Energy: 296 Kcal

Carbs: 41 g

Proteins: 9 g

Fats: 12 g

91. Vegan Quinoa and Avocado Salad

Preparation Time: 15 minutes

Cooking Time: 20 minutes

Portion Size: 2

Ingredients:

1/2 cup quinoa

1 avocado, diced

1 cup cherry tomatoes, halved

1/2 cup fresh spinach, chopped

1 tbsp olive oil

2 tbsp lemon juice

Salt and pepper to taste

Instructions:

Cook the quinoa according to package

Combine the cooked quinoa, diced avocado, cherry tomatoes, and chopped spinach in a large mixing basin.

In a small mixing bowl, combine the olive oil, lemon juice, salt, and pepper.

Toss the salad with the dressing to mix.

Serve immediately or refrigerate until ready to serve.

Nutrition Facts (1 portion):

Energy: 418 Kcal

Carbs: 46 g

Proteins: 10 g

Fats: 23 g

92. Vegan Stuffed Zucchini

Preparation Time: 15 minutes

Cooking Time: 25 minutes

Portion Size: 2 servings

Ingredients:

2 medium zucchinis

1 tablespoon olive oil

1 small onion, diced

2 cloves garlic, minced

1 medium tomato, diced

1 cup cooked quinoa

1/2 cup canned black beans, drained and rinsed

1/2 teaspoon ground cumin

1/2 teaspoon paprika

Salt and black pepper to taste

2 tablespoons chopped fresh parsley

Instructions:

Preheat the oven to 400°F (200°C).

Cut the zucchinis in half lengthwise and scoop out the meat, leaving a 1/4-inch thick shell on the outside.

In a pan over medium heat, heat the olive oil.

Sauté the onion and garlic until tender.

Add the tomato, quinoa, black beans, cumin, paprika, salt, and pepper to taste. Cook for a few minutes more, or until everything is thoroughly blended.

Fill the zucchini shells with the mixture.

Place the packed zucchinis on a baking sheet and bake for approximately 15-20 minutes, or until soft.

Sprinkle with chopped parsley before serving.

Nutrition Facts (1 serving):

Energy: 285 Kcal

Carbs: 37 g

Proteins: 11 g

Fats: 10 g

93. Vegan Vegetable Fried Rice

Preparation Time: 10 minutes

Cooking Time: 15 minutes

Portion Size: 2

Ingredients:

1 cup cooked brown rice

1/2 cup frozen mixed vegetables

1/2 onion, diced

1 clove garlic, minced

2 tbsp low-sodium soy sauce

1 tbsp olive oil

Instructions:

Heat the olive oil in a pan over medium heat.

Add the onion and garlic, sauté until onion is translucent.

Add the frozen mixed vegetables, cook until heated through.
Add the cooked brown rice and soy sauce, stir to combine.
Serve hot.

Nutrition Facts (1 portion):
Energy: 255 Kcal
Carbs: 44 g
Proteins: 6 g
Fats: 7 g

94. Vegan Zucchini Noodles with Tomato Sauce

Preparation Time: 15 minutes
Cooking Time: 10 minutes
Portion Size: 2

Ingredients:
2 medium zucchini
1 cup tomato sauce
1 clove garlic, minced
1 tbsp olive oil
Salt and pepper to taste

Instructions*:*
Use a spiralizer or a vegetable peeler to make zucchini noodles.
In a medium saucepan, heat the olive oil.
Sauté the garlic until fragrant.
Cook for 2-3 minutes, or until the zucchini noodles are soft.
Season with salt and pepper and whisk in the tomato sauce.
Serve hot.

Nutrition Facts (1 portion):
Energy: 141 Kcal
Carbs: 15 g
Proteins: 5 g
Fats: 8 g

95. Vegan Chickpea Salad

Preparation Time: 15 minutes
Cooking Time: 0 minutes
Portion Size: 2

Ingredients:
1 cup chickpeas, rinsed and drained
1 cucumber, diced
1 bell pepper, diced
1/4 cup fresh parsley, chopped
1 tbsp olive oil
2 tbsp lemon juice
Salt and pepper to taste

Instructions:
In a large bowl, combine the chickpeas, cucumber, bell pepper, and parsley.
In a small mixing bowl, combine the olive oil, lemon juice, salt, and pepper.
Toss the salad with the dressing to mix.
Refrigerate until ready to serve or serve immediately.

Nutrition Facts (1 portion):
Energy: 238 Kcal
Carbs: 32 g
Proteins: 9 g
Fats: 10 g

96. Vegan Pumpkin Soup

Preparation Time: 10 minutes
Cooking Time: 25 minutes
Portion Size: 2

Ingredients:
1 cup pumpkin puree
1 cup vegetable broth

1/2 onion, diced
1 clove garlic, minced
1/2 teaspoon cumin
1 tablespoon olive oil
Salt and pepper to taste

Instructions:

Heat the olive oil in a saucepan over medium heat.
Sauté the onion and garlic until the onion is transparent.
Combine the pumpkin puree, vegetable broth, cumin, salt, and pepper in a mixing bowl. To blend, stir everything together.
Bring to a boil, then lower to a low heat and cook for 20 minutes.
Serve hot.

Nutrition Facts (1 portion):

Energy: 133 Kcal
Carbs: 18 g
Proteins: 2 g
Fats: 7 g

97. Vegan Couscous Salad

Preparation Time: 10 minutes
Cooking Time: 5 minutes
Portion Size: 2

Ingredients:

1/2 cup couscous
1 cup vegetable broth
1 cucumber, diced
1/2 bell pepper, diced
1/4 cup fresh mint, chopped
2 tablespoons olive oil
1 tablespoon lemon juice
Salt and pepper to taste

Instructions:

In a saucepan, bring the vegetable broth to a boil.
Cover and remove from heat after adding the couscous. Allow to stand for 5 minutes before fluffing with a fork.
Combine the couscous, cucumber, bell pepper, and mint in a large mixing basin.
In a small mixing bowl, combine the olive oil, lemon juice, salt, and pepper.
Toss the salad with the dressing to mix.
Serve immediately or refrigerate until ready to serve.

Nutrition Facts (1 portion):

Energy: 253 Kcal
Carbs: 33 g
Proteins: 6 g
Fats: 11 g

98. Vegan Coconut Curry

Preparation Time: 10 minutes
Cooking Time: 20 minutes
Portion Size: 2

Ingredients:

1/2 cup canned chickpeas, rinsed and drained
1/2 can coconut milk
1/2 onion, diced
1 clove garlic, minced
1/2 bell pepper, diced
1 teaspoon curry powder
1 tablespoon olive oil
Salt to taste

Instructions:

Heat the olive oil in a pan over medium heat.
Add the onion, garlic, and bell pepper, sauté until onion is translucent.

Add the curry powder, stir to coat the vegetables.
Add the chickpeas and coconut milk, stir to combine.
Bring to a boil, then reduce heat and simmer for 15 minutes.
Serve hot, over brown rice if desired.

Nutrition Facts (1 portion):
Energy: 350 Kcal
Carbs: 28 g
Proteins: 8 g
Fats: 24 g

99. Vegan Berry Smoothie

Preparation Time: 5 minutes
Cooking Time: 0 minutes
Portion Size: 2

Ingredients:
1 banana
1 cup mixed berries, fresh or frozen
1 cup almond milk
1 tablespoon chia seeds

Instructions:
Combine all ingredients in a blender.
Blend until smooth.
Serve immediately.

Nutrition Facts (1 portion):
Energy: 158 Kcal
Carbs: 31 g
Proteins: 3 g
Fats: 4 g

100. Vegan Mushroom and Kale Pasta

Preparation Time: 10 minutes
Cooking Time: 20 minutes
Portion Size: 2

Ingredients:
2 cups whole wheat pasta
1 cup sliced mushrooms
1 cup kale, stems removed and leaves torn
1/2 onion, diced
1 clove garlic, minced
1 tablespoon olive oil
Salt and pepper to taste

Instructions:
Cook the pasta according to package
In a pan, heat the olive oil over medium heat.
Add the onion and garlic, sauté until onion is translucent.
Add the mushrooms, cook until browned.
Add the kale, cook until wilted.
Add the cooked pasta, season with salt and pepper, and stir to combine.
Serve hot.

Nutrition Facts (1 portion):
Energy: 376 Kcal
Carbs: 65 g
Proteins: 15 g
Fats: 8 g

101. Vegan Avocado Toast

Preparation Time: 5 minutes
Cooking Time: 5 minutes
Portion Size: 2

Ingredients:
2 slices of whole grain bread
1 ripe avocado
1/2 lemon, juiced
Salt and pepper to taste
Red pepper flakes (optional)

Instructions:

Toast the bread slices until golden brown.
Mash the avocado in a bowl, mix in lemon juice, salt, and pepper.
Spread the mashed avocado onto the toasted bread.
Sprinkle with red pepper flakes if desired.
Serve immediately.

Nutrition Facts (1 portion):

Energy: 233 Kcal
Carbs: 26 g
Proteins: 7 g
Fats: 13 g

102. Vegan Bulgur Salad

Preparation Time: 15 minutes
Cooking Time: 15 minutes
Portion Size: 2

Ingredients:

1 cup bulgur
2 cups water
1/2 cucumber, diced
1 medium tomato, diced
1/2 red onion, finely chopped
1/4 cup fresh parsley, finely chopped
1/4 cup fresh mint, finely chopped
2 tablespoons olive oil
Juice of 1 lemon
Salt and pepper to taste

Instructions:

Bring the water to a boil in a pot, add the bulgur and a pinch of salt. Reduce the heat to low, cover, and cook for 15 minutes, or until the water has been absorbed and the bulgur is soft.
When the bulgur has finished cooking, fluff it with a fork and set it aside to cool to room temperature.
Combine the chilled bulgur, cucumber, tomato, onion, parsley, and mint in a large mixing dish.
In a small mixing bowl, combine the olive oil, lemon juice, salt, and pepper. Pour the dressing over the salad and toss to combine.
Serve the salad immediately, or cover and chill for at least 1 hour to allow the flavors to mingle.

Nutrition Facts (1 portion):

Energy: 260 Kcal
Carbs: 50 g
Proteins: 6 g
Fats: 7 g

103. Vegan Banana Pancakes

Preparation Time: 5 minutes
Cooking Time: 10 minutes
Portion Size: 2

Ingredients:

1 ripe banana
1/2 cup oat flour
1/2 cup almond milk
1 teaspoon baking powder
1/2 teaspoon vanilla extract

Instructions:

Mash the banana in a bowl.
Add the oat flour, almond milk, baking powder, and vanilla extract. Stir to combine.
Heat a non-stick pan over medium heat.
Pour 1/4 of the batter onto the pan, cook until bubbles appear on the surface, then flip and cook the other side.
Repeat with the rest of the batter.

Serve hot, with your favorite fruit or syrup.

Nutrition Facts (1 portion):

Energy: 175 Kcal

Carbs: 35 g

Proteins: 4 g

Fats: 3 g

104. Vegan Spicy Tofu Stir-Fry

Preparation Time: 10 minutes

Cooking Time: 15 minutes

Portion Size: 2

Ingredients:

1/2 block firm tofu, drained and cut into cubes

1/2 bell pepper, sliced

1/2 onion, sliced

1 clove garlic, minced

1/2 teaspoon chili flakes

1 tablespoon soy sauce

1 tablespoon olive oil

Instructions:

Heat the olive oil in a pan over medium heat.

Add the tofu cubes, cook until browned on all sides.

Add the onion, bell pepper, garlic, and chili flakes. Stir-fry until vegetables are tender.

Add the soy sauce, stir to combine.

Serve hot, over brown rice if desired.

Nutrition Facts (1 portion):

Energy: 203 Kcal

Carbs: 9 g

Proteins: 11 g

Fats: 14 g

105. Vegan Berry Oatmeal

Preparation Time: 5 minutes

Cooking Time: 10 minutes

Portion Size: 2

Ingredients:

1 cup oats

2 cups almond milk

1 cup mixed berries, fresh or frozen

1 tablespoon maple syrup

Instructions:

In a saucepan, bring the almond milk to a boil.

Add the oats, reduce heat to low, and simmer for 10 minutes, stirring occasionally.

Stir in the berries and maple syrup.

Serve hot.

Nutrition Facts (1 portion):

Energy: 269 Kcal

Carbs: 47 g

Proteins: 7 g

Fats: 7 g

106. Vegan Chickpea Curry

Preparation Time: 5 minutes

Cooking Time: 20 minutes

Portion Size: 2

Ingredients:

1 can of chickpeas, drained and rinsed

1/2 can of diced tomatoes

1/2 onion, diced

1 clove garlic, minced

1/2 tsp curry powder

1/2 tsp turmeric

1 tbsp olive oil

Salt to taste

Instructions:

In a pan, heat olive oil over medium heat.
Add the onion and garlic, sauté until fragrant.
Add the chickpeas, diced tomatoes, curry powder, turmeric, and salt.
Simmer for 15-20 minutes until the flavors are well combined.
Serve warm with whole grain bread or rice.

Nutrition Facts (1 portion):
Energy: 312 Kcal
Carbs: 43 g
Proteins: 11 g
Fats: 12 g

107. Vegan Stuffed Bell Peppers

Preparation Time: 10 minutes
Cooking Time: 25 minutes
Portion Size: 2

Ingredients:
1 bell pepper, halved
1/2 cup cooked quinoa
1/2 can of black beans, rinsed and drained
1/2 cup corn
1/2 tsp chili powder
1/2 tsp cumin
Salt to taste

Instructions:
Preheat the oven to 375°F (190°C).
In a bowl, mix together the quinoa, black beans, corn, chili powder, cumin, and salt.
Scoop the mixture into the bell pepper halves.
Bake for 20-25 minutes until the peppers are tender.
Serve warm.

Nutrition Facts (1 portion):
Energy: 214 Kcal
Carbs: 42 g
Proteins: 10 g
Fats: 3 g

108. Vegan Split Pea Soup

Preparation Time: 15 minutes
Cooking Time: 45 minutes
Portion Size: 2

Ingredients:
1 cup split peas, rinsed
1 medium carrot, diced
1 celery stalk, diced
1/2 onion, diced
2 garlic cloves, minced
4 cups vegetable broth
1 bay leaf
Salt and pepper to taste
1 tablespoon olive oil

Instructions:
Heat the olive oil in a large pot over medium heat. Add the onion, carrot, celery, and garlic and sauté until the onions are translucent, about 5 minutes.
Add the split peas, vegetable broth, bay leaf, salt, and pepper to the pot. Bring to a boil, then lower to a low heat, cover, and let to cook for 45 minutes, or until the split peas are cooked.
Take out the bay leaf. Puree the soup with an immersion blender until smooth, or transfer to a countertop blender in stages and puree until smooth.
If required, adjust the spice before serving the soup hot.

Nutrition Facts (1 portion):
Energy: 365 Kcal
Carbs: 65 g

Proteins: 25 g

Fats: 5 g

109. Vegan Almond Butter Strawberry Smoothie

Preparation Time: 10 minutes

Portion Size: 2 servings

Ingredients:

2 ripe bananas

1 cup frozen strawberries

2 tablespoons almond butter

1 cup unsweetened almond milk

1 teaspoon chia seeds (optional)

Instructions:

Place bananas, frozen strawberries, almond butter, and almond milk into a blender.

Blend until the mixture is smooth and creamy. Add a bit more almond milk and mix again if the smoothie is too thick.

Pour the smoothie into two glasses.

Serve immediately, topped with chia seeds (if using).

Consider adding a scoop of your favorite plant-based protein powder for a protein boost.

Nutrition Facts (1 serving):

Energy: 240 Kcal

Carbs: 34 g

Proteins: 6 g

Fats: 10 g

110. Vegan Roasted Brussels Sprouts

Preparation Time: 5 minutes

Cooking Time: 20 minutes

Portion Size: 2

Ingredients:

2 cups Brussels sprouts, halved

1 tbsp olive oil

Salt and pepper to taste

Instructions:

Preheat the oven to 400°F (200°C).

Toss the Brussels sprouts with olive oil, salt, and pepper.

Spread them out on a baking sheet.

Roast for 20 minutes until golden and crispy.

Serve warm.

Nutrition Facts (1 portion):

Energy: 118 Kcal

Carbs: 11 g

Proteins: 4 g

Fats: 7 g

Snack

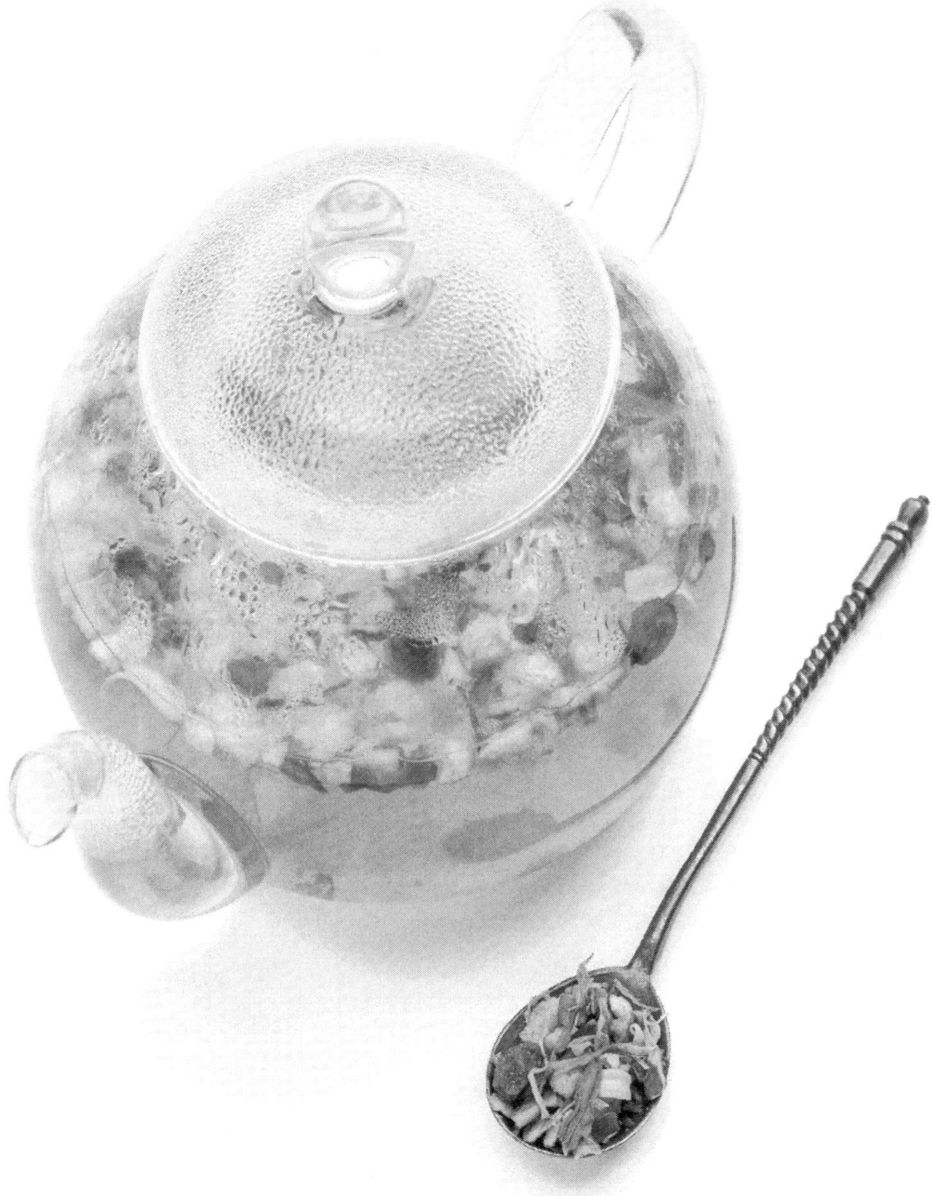

111. Zesty Lemon & Ginger Tea

Preparation Time: 5 minutes
Cooking Time: 10 minutes
Portion Size: 2

Ingredients:

2 cups water
2 slices of fresh ginger
Juice of 1 lemon
2 tsp honey

Instructions:

Boil water with ginger slices.
Remove from heat, add lemon juice and honey. Stir until honey is dissolved.
Serve immediately.

Nutrition Facts (1 portion):

Energy: 45 Kcal
Carbs: 12 g
Proteins: 0 g
Fats: 0 g

112. Avocado & Pomegranate Bruschetta

Preparation Time: 15 minutes
Portion Size: 2

Ingredients:

4 slices of whole grain bread
1 ripe avocado
1/2 cup pomegranate seeds
2 tablespoons of olive oil
Salt and pepper to taste

Instructions:

Toast the bread slices.
Meanwhile, halve the avocado, remove the seed and scoop out the flesh. Mash it in a bowl.
Spread the mashed avocado evenly onto the toasted bread slices.
Sprinkle pomegranate seeds over the avocado spread.
Drizzle with olive oil and season with salt and pepper.
Serve immediately.

Nutrition Facts (1 portion):

Energy: 300 Kcal
Carbs: 32 g
Proteins: 7 g
Fats: 17 g

113. Quick Veggie Stir-Fry

Preparation Time: 5 minutes
Cooking Time: 10 minutes
Portion Size: 2

Ingredients:

1 bell pepper, sliced
1 medium zucchini, sliced
1 tbsp olive oil
1 tbsp soy sauce

Instructions:

Heat olive oil in a pan over medium heat.
Add bell pepper and zucchini, stir-fry for 5 minutes.
Add soy sauce, stir well, and cook for another 5 minutes.
Serve immediately.

Nutrition Facts (1 portion):

Energy: 128 Kcal
Carbs: 9 g
Proteins: 3 g

Fats: 10 g

114. Fruit & Nut Energy Bars

Preparation Time: 10 minutes
Cooking Time: 0 minutes
Portion Size: 2

Ingredients:

1/2 cup pitted dates
1/2 cup walnuts
1/2 cup dried cranberries

Instructions:

Blend dates, walnuts, and cranberries in a food processor until they form a sticky mixture.
Press the mixture into a small pan or dish.
Refrigerate for 30 minutes, then cut into bars.

Nutrition Facts (1 portion):

Energy: 385 Kcal
Carbs: 50 g
Proteins: 8 g
Fats: 20 g

115. Baked Kale Chips

Preparation Time: 5 minutes
Cooking Time: 20 minutes
Portion Size: 2

Ingredients:

4 cups kale, torn into pieces
1 tbsp olive oil
A pinch of salt

Instructions:

Preheat your oven to 300°F (150°C).
Toss kale with olive oil and salt, spread out on a baking sheet.
Bake for 20 minutes or until crispy.
Serve immediately.

Nutrition Facts (1 portion):

Energy: 99 Kcal
Carbs: 8 g
Proteins: 4 g
Fats: 7 g

116. Sweet Potato Hummus

Preparation Time: 10 minutes
Cooking Time: 0 minutes
Portion Size: 2

Ingredients:

1 cup sweet potato, cooked and mashed
1/2 cup canned chickpeas, drained and rinsed
1 tbsp olive oil
1 tbsp lemon juice

Instructions:

Blend sweet potato, chickpeas, olive oil, and lemon juice in a food processor until smooth.
Serve immediately or refrigerate.

Nutrition Facts (1 portion):

Energy: 233 Kcal
Carbs: 38 g
Proteins: 6 g
Fats: 7 g

117. Cucumber & Avocado Salsa

Preparation Time: 10 minutes
Cooking Time: 0 minutes
Portion Size: 2

Ingredients:

1 cucumber, diced
1 ripe avocado, diced
1 tbsp olive oil
1 tbsp lemon juice
A pinch of salt

Instructions:

Combine cucumber and avocado in a bowl.
Drizzle with olive oil and lemon juice, sprinkle with salt, and toss to mix.
Serve immediately.

Nutrition Facts (1 portion):

Energy: 210 Kcal
Carbs: 12 g
Proteins: 3 g
Fats: 19 g

118. Papaya & Chia Pudding

Preparation Time: 15 minutes
Chilling Time: 2 hours or overnight
Portion Size: 2 servings

Ingredients:

1/2 cup chia seeds
1 cup almond milk (or any non-dairy milk)
1 small ripe papaya
1-2 tablespoons maple syrup or sweetener of choice (optional)
Fresh mint leaves for garnish (optional)

Instructions:

In a bowl, mix the chia seeds and almond milk. Stir well to combine and make sure there are no clumps.
Let the mixture sit for about 15 minutes until the chia seeds absorb the milk and the mixture becomes thick and pudding-like. You can also cover and refrigerate the mixture for a couple of hours or overnight for best results.
While the chia pudding is setting, cut the papaya in half lengthwise. Scoop out the seeds with a spoon and discard. Slice or cube the papaya flesh, as per your preference.
Once the chia pudding is ready, give it a stir and add sweetener if using. Adjust the consistency by adding a little more milk if it's too thick.
Divide the chia pudding into two serving bowls or glasses. Top each with papaya and garnish with mint leaves, if using.

Nutrition Facts (1 serving):

Energy: 220 Kcal
Carbs: 25 g
Proteins: 7 g
Fats: 11 g

119. Quinoa & Blueberry Muffins

Preparation Time: 10 minutes
Cooking Time: 20 minutes
Portion Size: 2

Ingredients:

1/2 cup cooked quinoa
1/2 cup almond flour
1/4 cup blueberries
2 tbsp honey
1/2 tsp baking powder

Instructions:

Preheat your oven to 350°F (175°C).
Combine all ingredients in a bowl, mix until combined.
Scoop into muffin cups and bake for 20 minutes or until golden.

Nutrition Facts (1 portion):

Energy: 225 Kcal
Carbs: 33 g
Proteins: 8 g
Fats: 8 g

120. Almond & Turmeric Latte

Preparation Time: 5 minutes
Cooking Time: 5 minutes
Portion Size: 2

Ingredients:

2 cups almond milk
1 tsp turmeric
1 tsp honey

Instructions:

Heat almond milk in a saucepan over medium heat.
Stir in turmeric and honey, heat until hot but not boiling.
Serve immediately.

Nutrition Facts (1 portion):

Energy: 100 Kcal
Carbs: 11 g
Proteins: 1 g
Fats: 5 g

121. Banana & Almond Butter Toast

Preparation Time: 5 minutes
Cooking Time: 0 minutes
Portion Size: 2

Ingredients:

2 slices whole grain bread
2 tbsp almond butter
1 banana, sliced

Instructions:

Spread almond butter evenly over each bread slice.
Top with banana slices.
Serve immediately.

Nutrition Facts (1 portion):

Energy: 250 Kcal
Carbs: 31 g
Proteins: 8 g
Fats: 13 g

122. Quinoa & Almond Energy Balls

Preparation Time: 15 minutes
Cooking Time: 0 minutes
Portion Size: 2

Ingredients:

1/2 cup cooked quinoa
1/2 cup dates, pitted
1/4 cup almonds
1 tbsp chia seeds

Instructions:

Blend all ingredients in a food processor until well combined.
Roll the mixture into balls.
Refrigerate for at least an hour before serving.

Nutrition Facts (1 portion):

Energy: 210 Kcal
Carbs: 32 g
Proteins: 5 g
Fats: 8 g

123. Avocado & Strawberry Bruschetta

Preparation Time: 15 minutes
Portion Size: 2

Ingredients:
2 slices of whole grain bread
1 ripe avocado
1 cup of fresh strawberries
1 tablespoon of fresh lemon juice
2 tablespoons of olive oil
Salt to taste
Freshly ground black pepper to taste
Fresh basil leaves for garnish (optional)

Instructions:
Toast the bread slices to your preferred level of crispiness.
Remove the pit from the avocado and scoop out the flesh. In a mixing dish, combine it with the lemon juice, salt, and pepper.
Wash the strawberries, remove the stems, and thinly slice them.
Evenly distribute the mashed avocado on the bread. Serve with strawberry slices on top.
Drizzle with olive oil and sprinkle with parsley, if using.
Serve immediately. Enjoy!

Nutrition Facts (1 portion):
Energy: 320 Kcal
Carbs: 27 g
Proteins: 6 g
Fats: 22 g

124. Spiced Pumpkin Seeds

Preparation Time: 5 minutes
Cooking Time: 10 minutes
Portion Size: 2

Ingredients:
1 cup pumpkin seeds
1/2 tsp olive oil
A pinch of salt
A pinch of cayenne pepper

Instructions:
Preheat your oven to 350°F (175°C).
Toss pumpkin seeds with olive oil, salt, and cayenne pepper.
Spread out on a baking sheet and bake for 10 minutes or until golden.

Nutrition Facts (1 portion):
Energy: 163 Kcal
Carbs: 3 g
Proteins: 7 g
Fats: 15 g

125. Mango & Coconut Smoothie

Preparation Time: 5 minutes
Cooking Time: 0 minutes
Portion Size: 2

Ingredients:
1 ripe mango, peeled and diced
1 cup coconut milk
1 tbsp honey

Instructions:
Blend all ingredients in a blender until smooth.
Serve immediately.

Nutrition Facts (1 portion):
Energy: 250 Kcal
Carbs: 30 g
Proteins: 2 g
Fats: 16 g

126. Green Tea & Honey Popsicles

Preparation Time: 5 minutes
Freezing Time: 4 hours
Portion Size: 2

Ingredients:
1 cup brewed green tea
2 tbsp honey

Instructions:
Mix the green tea and honey together until honey is dissolved.
Pour the mixture into popsicle molds.
Freeze for at least 4 hours before serving.

Nutrition Facts (1 portion):
Energy: 60 Kcal
Carbs: 17 g
Proteins: 0 g
Fats: 0 g

127. Baked Apple Chips

Preparation Time: 10 minutes
Cooking Time: 1 hour
Portion Size: 2

Ingredients:
2 apples, thinly sliced
1 tsp cinnamon

Instructions:
Preheat your oven to 200°F (93°C).
Spread the apple slices on a baking sheet and sprinkle with cinnamon.
Bake for 1 hour or until crispy, flipping the slices halfway.

Nutrition Facts (1 portion):
Energy: 95 Kcal
Carbs: 25 g
Proteins: 0.5 g
Fats: 0.3 g

128. Blueberry & Oat Bars

Preparation Time: 10 minutes
Cooking Time: 20 minutes
Portion Size: 2

Ingredients:
1/2 cup oats
1/2 cup fresh blueberries
2 tbsp honey
1 tbsp almond butter

Instructions:
Preheat your oven to 350°F (175°C).
Mix all ingredients together in a bowl.
Press the mixture into a small baking dish.
Bake for 20 minutes or until golden.
Let cool before cutting into bars.

Nutrition Facts (1 portion):
Energy: 160 Kcal
Carbs: 30 g
Proteins: 4 g
Fats: 4 g

129. Spicy Roasted Chickpeas

Preparation Time: 10 minutes
Cooking Time: 30 minutes
Portion Size: 2

Ingredients:
1 can chickpeas, drained and rinsed
1 tbsp olive oil
1/2 tsp chili powder
A pinch of salt

Instructions:
Preheat your oven to 400°F (200°C).

Toss the chickpeas with olive oil, chili powder, and salt.

Spread out on a baking sheet and bake for 30 minutes or until crispy.

Nutrition Facts (1 portion):

Energy: 190 Kcal

Carbs: 22 g

Proteins: 7 g

Fats: 9 g

130. Banana & Chia Seed Pudding

Preparation Time: 10 minutes

Chilling Time: 4 hours

Portion Size: 2

Ingredients:

1 banana, mashed

1 cup almond milk

2 tbsp chia seeds

1 tbsp honey

Instructions:

Mix all ingredients together in a bowl.

Chill in the refrigerator for at least 4 hours or until the chia seeds have absorbed the liquid and the mixture has a pudding-like consistency.

Nutrition Facts (1 portion):

Energy: 150 Kcal

Carbs: 28 g

Proteins: 4 g

Fats: 4 g

Bread

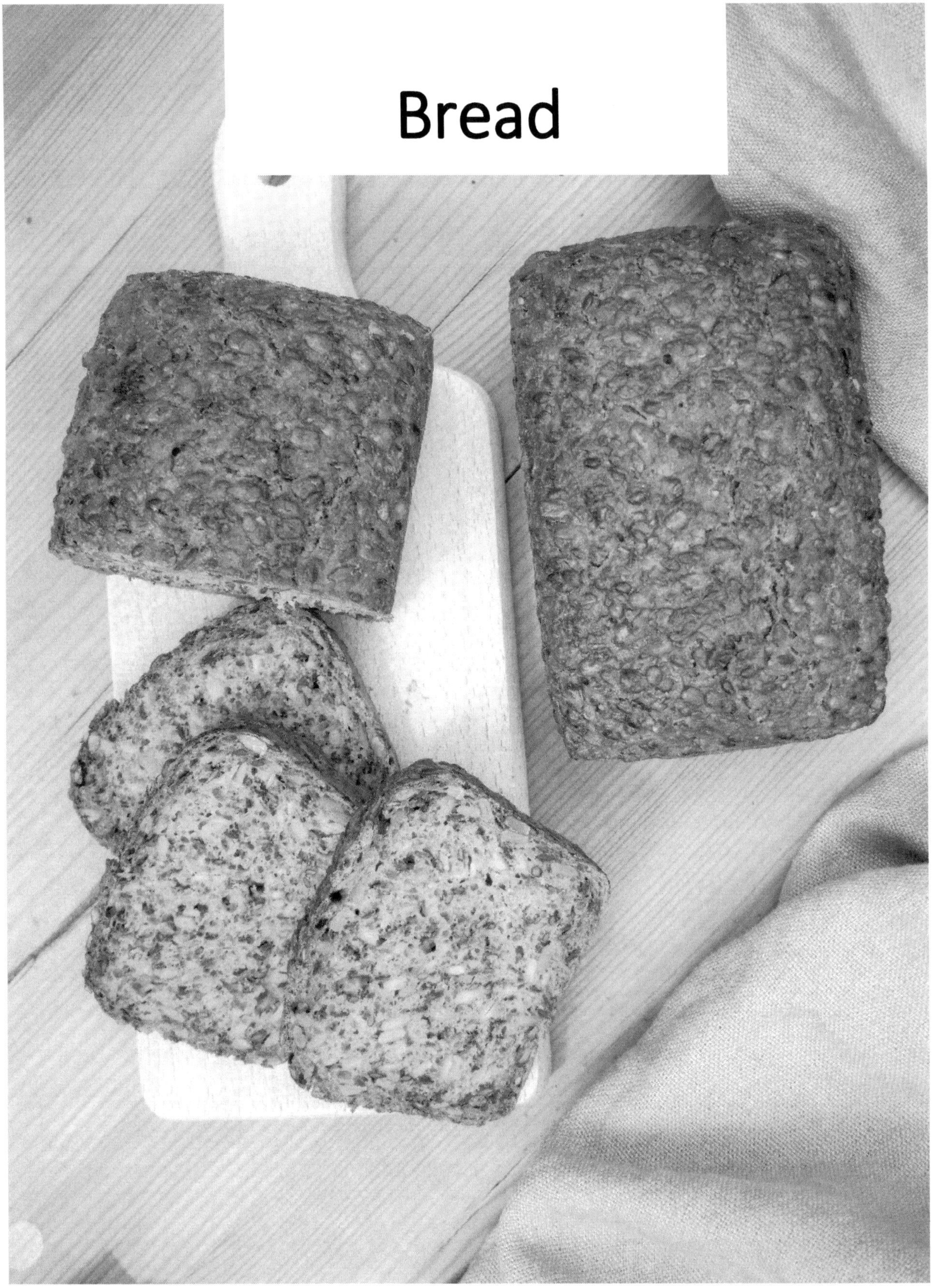

131. Brown Rice and Sesame Seed Bread

Preparation Time: 15 minutes
Cooking Time: 50 minutes
Portion Size: 2

Ingredients:

1 1/2 cups brown rice flour
1/2 cup sesame seeds
1 tsp baking powder
1/2 tsp salt
1 Tbsp olive oil
1 cup water

Instructions:

Preheat your oven to 350°F (180°C) and grease a loaf pan.
In a bowl, mix together the brown rice flour, sesame seeds, baking powder, and salt.
Add the olive oil and water. Stir until well combined.
Pour the batter into your prepared pan and bake for about 50 minutes, or until a toothpick inserted comes out clean.
Let the bread cool before slicing.

Nutrition Facts (1 portion):

Energy: 478 Kcal
Carbs: 68 g
Proteins: 12 g
Fats: 21 g

132. Almond and Flax Seed Bread

Preparation Time: 20 minutes + 30 minutes baking time
Portion Size: 2 servings

Ingredients:

1/3 cup almond flour
1 tablespoon flaxseed meal
1/3 tsp baking powder
A pinch of sea salt
1 large egg
2 tablespoons unsweetened almond milk
1 tsp olive oil

Instructions:

Preheat your oven to 350°F (175°C). Line a small loaf pan or muffin tin with parchment paper.
Combine the almond flour, flaxseed meal, baking powder, and sea salt in a mixing dish.
In a separate dish, combine the egg, almond milk, and olive oil.
Stir the dry ingredients into the wet components until the mixture is smooth.
Fill the loaf pan or muffin tray halfway with the batter.
Bake for 15-20 minutes, or until a toothpick inserted into the middle comes out clean.
Allow the bread to cool completely before slicing and serving. Serve it plain, toasted, or as the foundation for your favorite sandwich.

Nutrition Facts (1 portion):

Energy: 245 Kcal
Carbs: 6 g
Proteins: 10 g
Fats: 21 g

133. Spelt and Sunflower Seed Bread

Preparation Time: 10 minutes
Cooking Time: 60 minutes
Portion Size: 2

Ingredients:

1 1/2 cups spelt flour
1/2 cup sunflower seeds
1 tsp baking powder

1/2 tsp salt
1 Tbsp olive oil
1 cup water

Instructions:

Preheat your oven to 350°F (180°C) and grease a loaf pan.
In a bowl, mix together the spelt flour, sunflower seeds, baking powder, and salt.
Add the olive oil and water. Stir until well combined.
Pour the batter into your prepared pan and bake for about 60 minutes, or until a toothpick inserted comes out clean.
Let the bread cool before slicing.

Nutrition Facts (1 portion):

Energy: 473 Kcal
Carbs: 59 g
Proteins: 16 g
Fats: 22 g

134. Millet and Poppy Seed Bread

Preparation Time: 10 minutes
Cooking Time: 50 minutes
Portion Size: 2

Ingredients:

1 1/2 cups millet flour
1/2 cup poppy seeds
1 tsp baking powder
1/2 tsp salt
1 Tbsp olive oil
1 cup water

Instructions:

Preheat your oven to 350°F (180°C) and grease a loaf pan.
In a mixing dish, combine the millet flour, poppy seeds, baking powder, and salt.
Pour in the olive oil and water. Stir until well blended.
Pour the batter into the prepared pan and bake for 50 minutes, or until a toothpick inserted into the center comes out clean.
Let the bread cool before slicing.

Nutrition Facts (1 portion):

Energy: 469 Kcal
Carbs: 67 g
Proteins: 13 g
Fats: 19 g

135. Quinoa and Pumpkin Seed Bread

Preparation Time: 2 hours 15 minutes (including baking time)
Portion Size: 1 loaf (approximately 10 slices)

Ingredients:

1 cup quinoa
1/4 cup raw pumpkin seeds
1 1/2 cups water
1 tablespoon apple cider vinegar
1 tablespoon olive oil
1/2 teaspoon sea salt
1/2 teaspoon baking soda
1 tablespoon maple syrup (optional)

Instructions:

Rinse the quinoa under cold water until the water runs clear. Place the quinoa in a bowl, cover it with water, and let it soak for 1-2 hours.
Preheat your oven to 350°F (180°C). Line a loaf pan with parchment paper.
Place the quinoa in a blender and mix until smooth. Combine the pumpkin seeds, water, apple cider vinegar, olive oil, salt, baking soda, and maple syrup (if using) in a large mixing bowl. Blend until the batter is smooth.

Pour the batter into the loaf pan that has been prepared. Bake for 60-75 minutes, or until golden brown on top and a toothpick inserted into the middle comes out clean.

Allow the bread to cool for 15 minutes in the pan before transferring to a wire rack to cool entirely.

Slice and serve.

Note: This is a dense, hearty bread and is excellent for sandwiches or toast. Store in an airtight container for up to one week.

Nutrition Facts (1 slice):

Energy: 105 Kcal

Carbs: 15 g

Proteins: 4 g

Fats: 3 g

136. Buckwheat and Sunflower Seed Bread

Preparation Time: 2 hours 30 minutes (including resting and baking time)

Portion Size: 2 loaves

Ingredients:

3 cups buckwheat flour

1 cup sunflower seeds

1 1/2 cups warm water

2 tablespoons olive oil

2 tablespoons honey

1 packet (7 grams) of dry yeast

1 teaspoon salt

Instructions:

In a large bowl, combine the buckwheat flour and sunflower seeds.

In another bowl, dissolve the honey and yeast in warm water and let it sit for 5 minutes until foamy.

Pour the yeast and olive oil mixture into the flour mixture. Stir the dough until it comes together.

Knead the dough for approximately 10 minutes on a floured board, or until it is smooth and elastic.

Form the dough into a ball and return it to the bowl. Cover the bowl with a clean dish towel and let it aside for approximately 1 hour, or until it has doubled in size.

Punch the dough down and divide it into two equal portions when it has risen.

Place each component on a baking pan and shape it into a loaf. Allow the loaves to rest for 30 minutes, or until they puff up somewhat.

Preheat the oven to 375 degrees Fahrenheit (190 degrees Celsius).

Bake for 30-35 minutes, or until the loaves are golden brown and sound hollow when tapped on the bottom.

Let the loaves cool on a wire rack before slicing.

Nutrition Facts (1 slice):

Energy: 110 Kcal

Carbs: 18 g

Proteins: 4 g

Fats: 3 g

137. Amaranth and Sesame Seed Bread

Preparation Time: 10 minutes

Cooking Time: 50 minutes

Portion Size: 2

Ingredients:

1 1/2 cups amaranth flour

1/2 cup sesame seeds

1 tsp baking powder

1/2 tsp salt

1 Tbsp olive oil
1 cup water

Instructions:

Preheat your oven to 350°F (180°C) and grease a loaf pan.
In a mixing dish, combine the amaranth flour, sesame seeds, baking powder, and salt.
Pour in the olive oil and water. Stir until well blended.
Pour the batter into the prepared pan and bake for 50 minutes, or until a toothpick inserted into the center comes out clean.
Let the bread cool before slicing.

Nutrition Facts (1 portion):

Energy: 470 Kcal
Carbs: 58 g
Proteins: 13 g
Fats: 23 g

138. Millet and Flax Seed Bread

Preparation Time: 2 hours
Portion Size: 2 servings (around 8 slices)

Ingredients:

1 cup millet
2 tablespoons flax seeds
1 tablespoon olive oil
1/2 tablespoon yeast
1/2 tablespoon sugar
1/2 teaspoon salt
1 cup warm water

Instructions:

In a large bowl, combine millet and flax seeds.
In another bowl, dissolve yeast and sugar in warm water. Let it sit for 5 minutes until it becomes frothy.
Pour the yeast mixture into the millet and flax seeds. Mix in the olive oil and salt until fully blended.
Cover the bowl with a towel and let it aside for 1 hour, or until it has doubled in size.
Preheat the oven to 375 degrees Fahrenheit (190 degrees Celsius). Butter a loaf pan.
Place the loaf pan in the oven for 45 minutes, or until the bread is golden brown.
Remove from the oven and let it cool before slicing.

Nutrition Facts (1 portion):

Energy: 365 Kcal
Carbs: 62 g
Proteins: 11 g
Fats: 9 g

139. Pumpkin Seed Bread

Preparation Time: 10 minutes
Cooking Time: 50 minutes
Portion Size: 2

Ingredients:

1 1/2 cups teff flour
1/2 cup pumpkin seeds
1 tsp baking powder
1/2 tsp salt
1 Tbsp olive oil
1 cup water

Instructions:

Preheat your oven to 350°F (180°C) and grease a loaf pan.
In a mixing bowl, combine the teff flour, pumpkin seeds, baking powder, and salt.
Pour in the olive oil and water. Stir until well blended.

Pour the batter into the prepared pan and bake for 50 minutes, or until a toothpick inserted into the center comes out clean.
Let the bread cool before slicing.

Nutrition Facts (1 portion):
Energy: 490 Kcal
Carbs: 59 g
Proteins: 14 g
Fats: 24 g

140. Oat and Almond Bread

Preparation Time: 10 minutes
Cooking Time: 45 minutes
Portion Size: 2

Ingredients:
1 1/2 cups oat flour
1/2 cup almonds, chopped
1 tsp baking powder
1/2 tsp salt
1 Tbsp olive oil
1 cup water

Instructions:
Preheat your oven to 350°F (180°C) and grease a loaf pan.
In a mixing dish, combine the oat flour, chopped almonds, baking powder, and salt.
Pour in the olive oil and water. Stir until well blended.
Pour the batter into the prepared pan and bake for 45 minutes, or until a toothpick inserted into the center comes out clean.
Let the bread cool before slicing.

Nutrition Facts (1 portion):
Energy: 480 Kcal
Carbs: 56 g
Proteins: 13 g
Fats: 25 g

141. Spelt and Pumpkin Seed Bread

Preparation Time: 15 minutes
Cooking Time: 45 minutes
Portion Size: 2

Ingredients:
2 cups spelt flour
1 cup water
1 tablespoon dry yeast
1 teaspoon salt
2 tablespoons olive oil
1/2 cup pumpkin seeds

Instructions:
Preheat the oven to 375°F (190°C) and line a loaf pan with parchment paper.
Combine the spelt flour, yeast, and salt in a large mixing basin.
To the dry ingredients, add the water and olive oil and whisk until the dough comes together.
Fold the pumpkin seeds into the dough until they are equally distributed.
Allow the dough to rise for 15 minutes in the prepared loaf pan.
Bake for 45 minutes, or until the bread is golden brown and the bottom sounds hollow when tapped.
Let it cool before slicing.

Nutrition Facts (1 portion, about 2 slices):
Energy: 310 Kcal
Carbs: 46 g
Proteins: 12 g
Fats: 10 g

142. Sorghum and Walnut Bread

Preparation Time: 10 minutes

Cooking Time: 50 minutes
Portion Size: 2

Ingredients:
1 1/2 cups sorghum flour
1/2 cup walnuts, chopped
1 tsp baking powder
1/2 tsp salt
1 Tbsp olive oil
1 cup water

Instructions:
Preheat your oven to 350°F (180°C) and grease a loaf pan.
In a bowl, mix together the sorghum flour, chopped walnuts, baking powder, and salt.
Add the olive oil and water. Stir until well combined.
Pour the batter into your prepared pan and bake for about 50 minutes, or until a toothpick inserted comes out clean.
Let the bread cool before slicing.

Nutrition Facts (1 portion):
Energy: 510 Kcal
Carbs: 59 g
Proteins: 13 g
Fats: 28 g

143. Amaranth and Sunflower Seed Bread
Preparation Time: 20 minutes
Cooking Time: 40 minutes
Portion Size: 2

Ingredients:
1 cup spelt flour
1/2 cup amaranth flour
1/2 cup sunflower seeds
1 tsp salt
1 tsp baking soda
1 cup buttermilk
2 tbsp honey

Instructions:
Preheat your oven to 350°F (175°C) and grease a bread pan.
Combine the spelt flour, amaranth flour, sunflower seeds, salt, and baking soda in a large mixing basin.
In a separate dish, combine the buttermilk and honey and whisk until the honey is dissolved.
Pour in the wet ingredients and mix until just blended.
Bake for 40 minutes, or until a toothpick inserted into the middle comes out clean, in the prepared bread pan.
Let it cool before serving.

Nutrition Facts (1 portion):
Energy: 330 Kcal
Carbs: 48 g
Proteins: 11 g
Fats: 12 g

144. Millet and Sunflower Seed Bread
Preparation Time: 10 minutes
Cooking Time: 50 minutes
Portion Size: 2

Ingredients:
1 1/2 cups millet flour
1/2 cup sunflower seeds
1 tsp baking powder
1/2 tsp salt
1 Tbsp olive oil
1 cup water

Instructions:

Preheat your oven to 350°F (180°C) and grease a loaf pan.
Combine the millet flour, sunflower seeds, baking powder, and salt in a mixing dish.
Pour in the olive oil and water. Stir until well blended.
Pour the batter into the prepared pan and bake for 50 minutes, or until a toothpick inserted into the center comes out clean.
Let the bread cool before slicing.

Nutrition Facts (1 portion):
Energy: 505 Kcal
Carbs: 62 g
Proteins: 14 g
Fats: 26 g

145. Almond and Pumpkin Seed Bread

Preparation Time: 10 minutes
Cooking Time: 50 minutes
Portion Size: 2

Ingredients:
1 1/2 cups almond flour
1/2 cup pumpkin seeds
1 tsp baking powder
1/2 tsp salt
1 Tbsp olive oil
1 cup water

Instructions:
Preheat your oven to 350°F (180°C) and grease a loaf pan.
In a mixing dish, combine the almond flour, pumpkin seeds, baking powder, and salt.
Pour in the olive oil and water. Stir until well blended.
Pour the batter into the prepared pan and bake for 50 minutes, or until a toothpick inserted into the center comes out clean.
Let the bread cool before slicing.

Nutrition Facts (1 portion):
Energy: 520 Kcal
Carbs: 21 g
Proteins: 20 g
Fats: 44 g

146. Oat and Sesame Seed Bread

Preparation Time: 10 minutes
Cooking Time: 50 minutes
Portion Size: 2

Ingredients:
1 1/2 cups oat flour
1/2 cup sesame seeds
1 tsp baking powder
1/2 tsp salt
1 Tbsp olive oil
1 cup water

Instructions:
Preheat your oven to 350°F (180°C) and grease a loaf pan.
In a mixing dish, combine the oat flour, sesame seeds, baking powder, and salt.
Pour in the olive oil and water. Stir until well blended.
Pour the batter into the prepared pan and bake for 50 minutes, or until a toothpick inserted into the center comes out clean.
Let the bread cool before slicing.

Nutrition Facts (1 portion):
Energy: 500 Kcal
Carbs: 55 g
Proteins: 17 g
Fats: 28 g

147. Walnut and Flaxseed Bread

Preparation Time: 10 minutes
Cooking Time: 50 minutes
Portion Size: 2

Ingredients:

1 1/2 cups whole wheat flour
1/2 cup crushed walnuts
1/4 cup ground flaxseeds
1 tsp baking powder
1/2 tsp salt
1 Tbsp olive oil
1 cup water

Instructions:

Preheat your oven to 350°F (180°C) and grease a loaf pan.
Combine the whole wheat flour, smashed walnuts, ground flaxseeds, baking powder, and salt in a mixing bowl.
Pour in the olive oil and water. Stir until well blended.
Pour the batter into the prepared pan and bake for 50 minutes, or until a toothpick inserted into the center comes out clean.
Let the bread cool before slicing.

Nutrition Facts (1 portion):

Energy: 570 Kcal
Carbs: 61 g
Proteins: 19 g
Fats: 33 g

148. Rye and Chia Seed Bread

Preparation Time: 10 minutes
Cooking Time: 50 minutes
Portion Size: 2

Ingredients:

1 1/2 cups rye flour
1/4 cup chia seeds
1 tsp baking powder
1/2 tsp salt
1 Tbsp olive oil
1 cup water

Instructions:

Preheat your oven to 350°F (180°C) and grease a loaf pan.
In a mixing dish, combine the rye flour, chia seeds, baking powder, and salt.
Pour in the olive oil and water. Stir until well blended.
Pour the batter into the prepared pan and bake for 50 minutes, or until a toothpick inserted into the center comes out clean.
Let the bread cool before slicing.

Nutrition Facts (1 portion):

Energy: 535 Kcal
Carbs: 75 g
Proteins: 15 g
Fats: 24 g

149. Spelt and Poppy Seed Bread

Preparation Time: 10 minutes
Cooking Time: 50 minutes
Portion Size: 2

Ingredients:

1 1/2 cups spelt flour
1/4 cup poppy seeds
1 tsp baking powder
1/2 tsp salt
1 Tbsp olive oil
1 cup water

Instructions:

Preheat your oven to 350°F (180°C) and grease a loaf pan.

In a mixing basin, combine the spelt flour, poppy seeds, baking powder, and salt.

Pour in the olive oil and water. Stir until well blended.

Pour the batter into the prepared pan and bake for 50 minutes, or until a toothpick inserted into the center comes out clean.

Let the bread cool before slicing.

Nutrition Facts (1 portion):

Energy: 510 Kcal

Carbs: 70 g

Proteins: 18 g

Fats: 23 g

150. Quinoa and Flaxseed Bread

Preparation Time: 10 minutes

Cooking Time: 50 minutes

Portion Size: 2

Ingredients:

1 cup cooked quinoa

1/2 cup ground flaxseed

1 cup whole wheat flour

1 tsp baking powder

1/2 tsp salt

1 Tbsp olive oil

1/2 cup water

Instructions:

Preheat your oven to 350°F (180°C) and grease a loaf pan.

Combine the cooked quinoa, ground flaxseed, whole wheat flour, baking powder, and salt in a mixing bowl.

Pour in the olive oil and water. Stir until well blended.

Pour the batter into the prepared pan and bake for 50 minutes, or until a toothpick inserted into the center comes out clean.

Let the bread cool before slicing.

Nutrition Facts (1 portion):

Energy: 555 Kcal

Carbs: 72 g

Proteins: 20 g

Fats: 25 g

Dessert

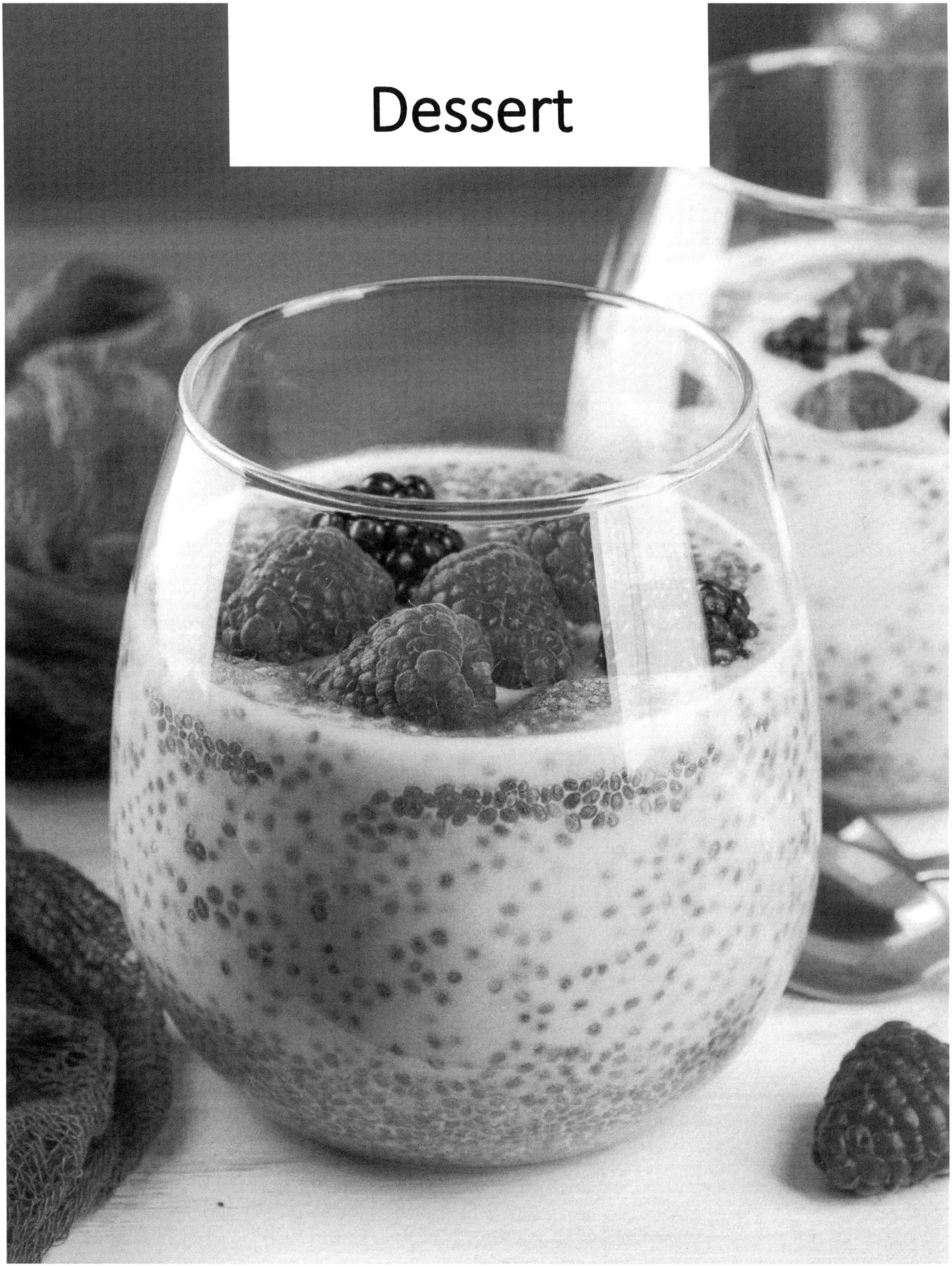

151. Raspberry Chia Pudding

Preparation Time: 5 minutes
Chill Time: 2 hours
Portion Size: 2

Ingredients:

1 cup fresh raspberries
1 cup almond milk, unsweetened
1/4 cup chia seeds
2 Tbsp honey
1/2 tsp vanilla extract
1/4 cup slivered almonds

Instructions:

Combine raspberries, almond milk, chia seeds, honey, and vanilla extract in a blender. Blend until smooth.
Pour the mixture into two glasses and refrigerate for at least 2 hours, or until it has a pudding-like consistency.
Before serving, sprinkle with slivered almonds.
Serve chilled.

Nutrition Facts (1 portion):

Energy: 200 Kcal
Carbs: 26 g
Proteins: 6 g
Fats: 9 g

152. Cocoa Banana Ice Cream

Preparation Time: 10 minutes
Freezing Time: 2 hours
Portion Size: 2

Ingredients:

2 ripe bananas
2 Tbsp unsweetened cocoa powder
1/4 cup almond milk, unsweetened
1 Tbsp honey
1/2 tsp vanilla extract

Instructions:

Peel bananas and slice them into small pieces. Freeze for at least 2 hours.
Blend frozen bananas, cocoa powder, almond milk, honey, and vanilla extract until smooth.
Serve immediately for a soft-serve consistency, or freeze for an additional hour for a firmer texture.

Nutrition Facts (1 portion):

Energy: 180 Kcal
Carbs: 42 g
Proteins: 3 g
Fats: 2 g

153. Blueberry Almond Tart

Preparation Time: 10 minutes
Cooking Time: 25 minutes
Portion Size: 2

Ingredients:

1/2 cup almond flour
2 Tbsp coconut oil, melted
1 Tbsp honey
1/2 cup fresh blueberries
1/4 tsp almond extract
1/4 cup sliced almonds

Instructions:

Preheat oven to 350°F (175°C). Combine almond flour, coconut oil, and honey in a

bowl, then press into the bottom of a small tart pan.
Bake for 10-15 minutes, until lightly golden.
Toss blueberries with almond extract, then spread over the crust. Sprinkle with sliced almonds.
Bake for an additional 10 minutes, until blueberries are juicy and almonds are toasted.
Cool completely before serving.

Nutrition Facts (1 portion):
Energy: 250 Kcal
Carbs: 15 g
Proteins: 5 g
Fats: 21 g

154. Peach Parfait
Preparation Time: 10 minutes
Chill Time: 0 minutes
Portion Size: 2

Ingredients:
2 peaches, pitted and diced
1 cup unsweetened Greek yogurt
1 Tbsp honey
1/4 cup granola
2 Tbsp chopped walnuts

Instructions:
Divide half of the peaches between two glasses. Layer with half of the Greek yogurt, honey, granola, and walnuts.
Repeat with the remaining ingredients.
Serve immediately

Nutrition Facts (1 portion):
Energy: 200 Kcal
Carbs: 27 g
Proteins: 12 g
Fats: 7 g

155. Strawberry Oat Bars
Preparation Time: 10 minutes
Cooking Time: 20 minutes
Portion Size: 2

Ingredients:
1/2 cup rolled oats
2 Tbsp almond butter
1 Tbsp honey
1/2 cup fresh strawberries, hulled and sliced
2 Tbsp chopped almonds

Instructions:
Preheat oven to 350°F (175°CIn a mixing dish, combine the oats, almond butter, and honey.
Half of the oat mixture should be pressed into the bottom of a small baking dish.
Top with the remaining oat mixture, then layer with strawberries and sliced almonds.
20 minutes, or until golden and set.
Allow to cool fully before slicing into bars.

Nutrition Facts (1 portion):
Energy: 240 Kcal
Carbs: 30 g
Proteins: 7 g
Fats: 12 g

156. Avocado Chocolate Mousse
Preparation Time: 10 minutes
Chill Time: 2 hours
Portion Size: 2

Ingredients:
1 ripe avocado
1/4 cup unsweetened cocoa powder

3 Tbsp honey
1/2 tsp vanilla extract
A pinch of salt

Instructions:
Blend all the ingredients in a blender or food processor until smooth.
Divide the mousse into two dessert cups and chill in the refrigerator for at least 2 hours.
Serve chilled.

Nutrition Facts (1 portion):
Energy: 210 Kcal
Carbs: 31 g
Proteins: 3 g
Fats: 11 g

157. Coconut Pineapple Sorbet

Preparation Time: 10 minutes + freezing time
Portion Size: 2 servings

Ingredients:
1/2 ripe pineapple, peeled, cored, and cut into chunks
1/2 can (200ml) of full-fat coconut milk
1/4 cup (50g) of granulated sugar
1/2 tablespoon of lime juice

Instructions:
In a blender or food processor, combine pineapple chunks, coconut milk, sugar, and lime juice. Blend until smooth.
Pour the mixture into a loaf pan or a shallow, freezer-safe dish.
Freeze for 1 hour, then remove from the freezer and stir with a fork to break up any large ice crystals.
Cover and freeze for an additional 2-3 hours, or until the sorbet is firm.
Before serving, let the sorbet sit out at room temperature for 5-10 minutes to make scooping easier.
Serve immediately for the best texture.

Nutrition Facts (1 portion):
Energy: 245 Kcal
Carbs: 35 g
Proteins: 2 g
Fats: 12 g

158. Pineapple Coconut Chia Pudding

Preparation Time: 5 minutes
Chill Time: 2 hours
Portion Size: 2

Ingredients:
1 cup unsweetened coconut milk
1/4 cup chia seeds
1 Tbsp honey
1 cup diced fresh pineapple
2 Tbsp shredded coconut, unsweetened

Instructions:
Mix coconut milk, chia seeds, and honey in a bowl. Divide the mixture into two glasses and chill in the refrigerator for at least 2 hours.
Top each pudding with pineapple and shredded coconut before serving.
Serve chilled.

Nutrition Facts (1 portion):
Energy: 220 Kcal
Carbs: 25 g
Proteins: 4 g
Fats: 12 g

159. Apple Cinnamon Baked Oatmeal Cups

Preparation Time: 10 minutes
Cooking Time: 20 minutes
Portion Size: 2

Ingredients:
1 cup rolled oats
1/2 cup diced apple
1/2 tsp cinnamon
1/2 cup almond milk, unsweetened
1 Tbsp honey

Instructions:
Preheat the oven to 350°F (175°C). Mix all the ingredients in a bowl.
Divide the mixture into a muffin tin to make two large oatmeal cups.
Bake for 20 minutes, or until golden.
Serve warm or at room temperature.

Nutrition Facts (1 portion):
Energy: 220 Kcal
Carbs: 43 g
Proteins: 6 g
Fats: 4 g

160. Berry Almond Crumble

Preparation Time: 10 minutes
Cooking Time: 30 minutes
Portion Size: 2

Ingredients:
1 cup mixed berries (like blueberries, raspberries, strawberries)
2 Tbsp honey, divided
1/2 cup rolled oats
1/4 cup almond meal
2 Tbsp coconut oil, melted

Instructions:
Preheat the oven to 350°F (175°C). Toss the berries with 1 Tbsp of honey and put them in a small baking dish.
In another bowl, mix oats, almond meal, coconut oil, and remaining honey. Sprinkle this mixture over the berries.
Bake for 30 minutes, or until the top is golden and the berries are bubbly.
Serve warm.

Nutrition Facts (1 portion):
Energy: 320 Kcal
Carbs: 36 g
Proteins: 7 g
Fats: 18 g

161. Spiced Baked Apples

Preparation Time: 10 minutes
Cooking Time: 30 minutes
Portion Size: 2

Ingredients:
2 apples
1/4 cup walnuts, chopped
2 Tbsp honey
1/2 tsp cinnamon
1/4 tsp nutmeg

Instructions:
Preheat the oven to 350°F (175°C). Core the apples and place them in a baking dish.
In a small bowl, mix the walnuts, honey, cinnamon, and nutmeg. Spoon this mixture into the hollowed-out cores of the apples.
Bake for 30 minutes, or until the apples are tender.
Serve warm.
Nutrition Facts (1 portion):
Energy: 195 Kcal
Carbs: 35 g

Proteins: 2 g
Fats: 7 g

162. Berry Quinoa Pudding

Preparation Time: 5 minutes
Cooking Time: 25 minutes
Portion Size: 2

Ingredients:

1/2 cup quinoa, rinsed
1 cup almond milk, unsweetened
1/4 cup mixed berries (fresh or frozen)
2 Tbsp honey
1/4 tsp vanilla extract

Instructions:

Combine the quinoa and almond milk in a saucepan. Bring to a boil, then reduce heat to low, cover, and simmer for 15 minutes, or until the quinoa is tender.
Stir in the mixed berries, honey, and vanilla extract. Cook for another 5-10 minutes, until the berries are soft and the mixture is thick and creamy.
Serve warm or chilled.

Nutrition Facts (1 portion):

Energy: 265 Kcal
Carbs: 50 g
Proteins: 7 g
Fats: 4 g

163. Coconut Mango Sorbet

Preparation Time: 10 minutes
Freezing Time: 2 hours
Portion Size: 2

Ingredients:

1 ripe mango, peeled and pitted
1/2 cup coconut milk, canned
2 Tbsp honey

Instructions:

Blend the mango, coconut milk, and honey in a blender until smooth.
Pour the mixture into a shallow dish and freeze for at least 2 hours.
Before serving, let it sit at room temperature for a few minutes to soften slightly.
Serve scoops of sorbet in dessert dishes.

Nutrition Facts (1 portion):

Energy: 180 Kcal
Carbs: 35 g
Proteins: 2 g
Fats: 6 g

164. Cherry Almond Clusters

Preparation Time: 10 minutes
Chill Time: 30 minutes
Portion Size: 2

Ingredients:

1/2 cup dark chocolate chips (at least 70% cocoa)
1/4 cup dried cherries
1/4 cup raw almonds

Instructions:

Melt the chocolate chips in a microwave or over a double boiler. Stir until smooth.
Mix in the dried cherries and almonds, making sure they're completely coated with chocolate.
Spoon small mounds of the mixture onto a parchment-lined baking sheet. Chill in the refrigerator for 30 minutes, or until set.

Nutrition Facts (1 portion):

Energy: 315 Kcal
Carbs: 28 g
Proteins: 6 g
Fats: 21 g

165. Pineapple Ginger Smoothie

Preparation Time: 5 minutes
Chill Time: 0 minutes
Portion Size: 2

Ingredients:

1 cup pineapple chunks
1 cup almond milk, unsweetened
1 Tbsp fresh ginger, grated
1 Tbsp honey

Instructions:

Blend the pineapple chunks, almond milk, ginger, and honey in a blender until smooth.
Serve immediately in two glasses.

Nutrition Facts (1 portion):

Energy: 120 Kcal
Carbs: 26 g
Proteins: 1 g
Fats: 2 g

166. Banana Walnut Mini Muffins

Preparation Time: 10 minutes
Cooking Time: 15 minutes
Portion Size: 2

Ingredients:

1 ripe banana, mashed
1/2 cup oat flour
1/4 cup walnuts, chopped
1/4 cup maple syrup
1/2 tsp baking soda
1/4 tsp vanilla extract

Instructions:

Preheat the oven to 350°F (175°C). Grease a mini muffin tin.
In a bowl, combine all ingredients. Mix well.
Scoop the batter into the prepared muffin tin.
Bake for 15 minutes, or until a toothpick inserted into the center of a muffin comes out clean.
Allow to cool before serving.

Nutrition Facts (1 portion):

Energy: 330 Kcal
Carbs: 49 g
Proteins: 7 g
Fats: 14 g

167. Chia Pudding with Blueberries

Preparation Time: 5 minutes
Chill Time: 2 hours
Portion Size: 2

Ingredients:

1/4 cup chia seeds
1 cup almond milk, unsweetened
1 Tbsp honey
1/2 cup fresh blueberries

Instructions:

In a bowl, combine the chia seeds, almond milk, and honey. Stir well.
Cover the bowl and place it in the refrigerator for at least 2 hours, or until the mixture has thickened into a pudding-like consistency.
Serve the chia pudding topped with fresh blueberries.

Nutrition Facts (1 portion):

Energy: 230 Kcal
Carbs: 30 g
Proteins: 7 g
Fats: 11 g

168. Dark Chocolate Avocado Mousse

Preparation Time: 10 minutes
Chill Time: 1 hour
Portion Size: 2

Ingredients:

1 ripe avocado, peeled and pitted
1/4 cup dark cocoa powder
1/4 cup maple syrup
1/2 tsp vanilla extract

Instructions:

Blend all ingredients in a blender or food processor until smooth.
Transfer the mousse to two serving dishes and chill in the refrigerator for at least 1 hour before serving.

Nutrition Facts (1 portion):

Energy: 310 Kcal
Carbs: 47 g
Proteins: 5 g
Fats: 15 g

169. Roasted Peaches with Almond Butter Drizzle

Preparation Time: 10 minutes
Cooking Time: 20 minutes
Portion Size: 2

Ingredients:

2 peaches, halved and pitted
1 Tbsp coconut oil
2 Tbsp almond butter
1 Tbsp honey

Instructions:

Preheat the oven to 375°F (190°C). Brush the cut sides of the peaches with coconut oil and place them cut-side down on a baking sheet.
Roast for 20 minutes, or until the peaches are tender and slightly caramelized.
Drizzle with almond butter and honey before serving.

Nutrition Facts (1 portion):

Energy: 230 Kcal
Carbs: 29 g
Proteins: 5 g
Fats: 12 g

170. Frozen Berry Yogurt Bites

Preparation Time: 10 minutes
Freezing Time: 2 hours
Portion Size: 2

Ingredients:

1/2 cup Greek yogurt, unsweetened
1/2 cup mixed berries
1 Tbsp honey

Instructions:

Blend the yogurt and berries in a blender until smooth. Stir in the honey.
Spoon the mixture into a silicone mold or ice cube tray.
Freeze for at least 2 hours, or until firm.
Pop out the frozen bites and serve.

Nutrition Facts (1 portion):

Energy: 90 Kcal
Carbs: 14 g
Proteins: 7 g
Fats: 1 g

171. Cinnamon Apple Amaranth

Preparation Time: 5 minutes
Cooking Time: 25 minutes
Portion Size: 2 servings

Ingredients:

1/2 cup amaranth
2 cups water
1 large apple, cored and diced
1 teaspoon cinnamon
1 tablespoon maple syrup or sweetener of choice
1/2 teaspoon vanilla extract

Instructions:

Rinse the amaranth under cold water and drain.
In a medium-sized pot, bring the water to a boil. Add the rinsed amaranth and reduce the heat to low, letting it simmer.
Cook the amaranth uncovered for about 20 minutes until most of the water is absorbed.
While the amaranth is cooking, place the diced apple in a microwave-safe bowl and sprinkle with the cinnamon. Cover the bowl with a microwave-safe plate and microwave for 2-3 minutes, until the apple is soft.
Once the amaranth is ready, stir in the cooked apple, maple syrup, and vanilla extract.
Serve hot and enjoy this nutritious and comforting breakfast!
Nutrition Facts (1 serving):
Energy: 280 Kcal
Carbs: 56 g
Proteins: 7 g
Fats: 3.5 g

60 DAY MEAL PLAN

This 60-day meal plan provides you with a variety of breakfast, lunch, and dinner options, as well as snacks and desserts. Including a diverse selection of recipes in your diet can provide you with a variety of flavors and nutrients, promoting a well-rounded and delicious eating experience. It is important to keep in mind that adjusting portion sizes and ingredients to meet your individual dietary needs and preferences is crucial for maintaining a healthy and balanced diet. Combining all the recipes in this cookbook can make a 2000-day meal plan.

Day 1:

Breakfast: Almond Milk Oatmeal
Lunch: Greek Lentil Salad
Dinner: Greek Salad Wrap

Day 2:

Breakfast: Pineapple Kale Smoothie
Lunch: Veggie-Packed Lentil Soup
Dinner: Chickpea and Spinach Pasta

Day 3:

Breakfast: Tempeh Scramble
Lunch: Avocado Chicken Salad
Dinner: Spinach and Goat Cheese Omelette

Day 4:

Breakfast: Quinoa and Almond Porridge
Lunch: Shrimp and Broccoli Stir Fry
Dinner: Quinoa and Black Bean Salad

Day 5:

Breakfast: Mango Chia Pudding
Lunch: Salmon with Lemon-Dill Sauce
Dinner: Grilled Salmon with Asparagus

Day 6:

Breakfast: Green Tea Smoothie
Lunch: Rainbow Salad Wraps
Dinner: Pineapple & Tofu Stir-fry

Day 7:

Breakfast: Baked Avocado Eggs
Lunch: Mediterranean Quinoa Salad
Dinner: Shrimp Avocado Salad

Day 8:

Breakfast: Cinnamon Apple Quinoa
Lunch: Greek Lentil Salad
Dinner: Chicken & Broccoli Stir-fry

Day 9:

Breakfast: Berry Greek Yogurt Parfait
Lunch: Baked Sweet Potato
Dinner: Mediterranean Bulgur Salad

Day 10:

Breakfast: Sweet Potato Hash
Lunch: Avocado Egg Salad

Dinner: Garlic Shrimp with Zucchini Noodles

Day 11:

Breakfast: Strawberry Banana Oatmeal
Lunch: Turkey Lettuce Wraps
Dinner: Cauliflower Rice & Vegetables

Day 12:

Breakfast: Pineapple Spinach Smoothie
Lunch: Quinoa Salad with Fresh Veggies
Dinner: Ginger-Sesame Salmon

Day 13:

Breakfast: Almond Butter Toast with Blueberries
Lunch: Balsamic Grilled Chicken and Veggies
Dinner: Quinoa & Black Bean Tacos

Day 14:

Breakfast: Chia Berry Yogurt Parfait
Lunch: Avocado and Black Bean Tacos
Dinner: Zucchini & Yellow Squash Soup

Day 15:

Breakfast: Veggie Omelet
Lunch: Sweet Potato and Spinach Curry
Dinner: Greek Yogurt Chicken

Day 16:

Breakfast: Avocado Tuna Salad
Lunch: Turkey and Veggie Stir Fry
Dinner: Spaghetti Squash with Cherry Tomatoes

Day 17:

Breakfast: Overnight Apple Cinnamon Oats
Lunch: Veggie and Quinoa Stuffed Bell Peppers
Dinner: Lemon-Dill Grilled Shrimp

Day 18:

Breakfast: Blueberry Almond Milk Smoothie
Lunch: Butternut Squash Soup
Dinner: Mediterranean Tofu Stir-Fry

Day 19:

Breakfast: Tofu Scramble with Veggies
Lunch: Grilled Chicken and Veggie Skewers
Dinner: Baked Cod with Lemon & Parsley

Day 20:

Breakfast: Avocado and Tomato Open Sandwich
Lunch: Lentil Stew
Dinner: Quinoa Salad with Avocado & Cucumber

Day 21:

Breakfast: Almond Milk Oatmeal
Lunch: Greek Lentil Salad
Dinner: Greek Salad Wrap

Day 22:

Breakfast: Pineapple Kale Smoothie
Lunch: Veggie-Packed Lentil Soup
Dinner: Chickpea and Spinach Pasta

Day 23:

Breakfast: Tempeh Scramble

Lunch: Avocado Chicken Salad

Dinner: Spinach and Goat Cheese Omelette

Day 24:

Breakfast: Quinoa and Almond Porridge

Lunch: Shrimp and Broccoli Stir Fry

Dinner: Quinoa and Black Bean Salad

Day 25:

Breakfast: Mango Chia Pudding

Lunch: Salmon with Lemon-Dill Sauce

Dinner: Grilled Salmon with Asparagus

Day 26:

Breakfast: Green Tea Smoothie

Lunch: Rainbow Salad Wraps

Dinner: Pineapple & Tofu Stir-fry

Day 27:

Breakfast: Baked Avocado Eggs

Lunch: Mediterranean Quinoa Salad

Dinner: Shrimp Avocado Salad

Day 28:

Breakfast: Cinnamon Apple Quinoa

Lunch: Greek Lentil Salad

Dinner: Chicken & Broccoli Stir-fry

Day 29:

Breakfast: Berry Greek Yogurt Parfait

Lunch: Baked Sweet Potato

Dinner: Mediterranean Bulgur Salad

Day 30:

Breakfast: Sweet Potato Hash

Lunch: Avocado Egg Salad

Dinner: Garlic Shrimp with Zucchini Noodles

Day 31:

Breakfast: Strawberry Banana Oatmeal

Lunch: Turkey Lettuce Wraps

Dinner: Cauliflower Rice & Vegetables

Day 32:

Breakfast: Pineapple Spinach Smoothie

Lunch: Quinoa Salad with Fresh Veggies

Dinner: Ginger-Sesame Salmon

Day 33:

Breakfast: Almond Butter Toast with Blueberries

Lunch: Balsamic Grilled Chicken and Veggies

Dinner: Quinoa & Black Bean Tacos

Day 34:

Breakfast: Chia Berry Yogurt Parfait

Lunch: Avocado and Black Bean Tacos

Dinner: Zucchini & Yellow Squash Soup

Day 35:

Breakfast: Veggie Omelet

Lunch: Sweet Potato and Spinach Curry

Dinner: Greek Yogurt Chicken

Day 36:

Breakfast: Avocado Tuna Salad

Lunch: Turkey and Veggie Stir Fry

Dinner: Spaghetti Squash with Cherry Tomatoes

Day 37:

Breakfast: Overnight Apple Cinnamon Oats

Lunch: Veggie and Quinoa Stuffed Bell Peppers

Dinner: Lemon-Dill Grilled Shrimp

Day 38:

Breakfast: Blueberry Almond Milk Smoothie

Lunch: Butternut Squash Soup

Dinner: Mediterranean Tofu Stir-Fry

Day 39:

Breakfast: Tofu Scramble with Veggies

Lunch: Grilled Chicken and Veggie Skewers

Dinner: Baked Cod with Lemon & Parsley

Day 40:

Breakfast: Avocado and Tomato Open Sandwich

Lunch: Lentil Stew

Dinner: Quinoa Salad with Avocado & Cucumber

Day 41:

Breakfast: Quinoa and Almond Porridge

Lunch: Greek Lentil Salad

Dinner: Quinoa & Black Bean Tacos

Day 42:

Breakfast: Berry Greek Yogurt Parfait

Lunch: Veggie and Quinoa Stuffed Bell Peppers

Dinner: Mediterranean Tofu Stir-Fry

Day 43:

Breakfast: Almond Butter Toast with Blueberries

Lunch: Avocado Chicken Salad

Dinner: Ginger-Sesame Salmon

Day 44:

Breakfast: Green Tea Smoothie

Lunch: Mediterranean Quinoa Salad

Dinner: Cauliflower Rice & Vegetables

Day 45:

Breakfast: Avocado Tuna Salad

Lunch: Salmon with Lemon-Dill Sauce

Dinner: Greek Yogurt Chicken

Day 46:

Breakfast: Baked Avocado Eggs

Lunch: Rainbow Salad Wraps

Dinner: Spaghetti Squash with Cherry Tomatoes

Day 47:

Breakfast: Sweet Potato Hash

Lunch: Greek Lentil Salad

Dinner: Lemon-Dill Grilled Shrimp

Dinner: Spinach and Goat Cheese Omelette

Day 48:

Breakfast: Cinnamon Apple Quinoa

Lunch: Baked Sweet Potato

Dinner: Baked Cod with Lemon & Parsley

Day 49:

Breakfast: Almond Milk Oatmeal

Lunch: Avocado Egg Salad

Dinner: Quinoa Salad with Avocado & Cucumber

Day 50:

Breakfast: Mango Chia Pudding

Lunch: Turkey Lettuce Wraps

Dinner: Mediterranean Bulgur Salad

Day 51:

Breakfast: Overnight Apple Cinnamon Oats

Lunch: Quinoa Salad with Fresh Veggies

Dinner: Greek Salad Wrap

Day 52:

Breakfast: Blueberry Almond Milk Smoothie

Lunch: Balsamic Grilled Chicken and Veggies

Dinner: Chickpea and Spinach Pasta

Day 53:

Breakfast: Tofu Scramble with Veggies

Lunch: Avocado and Black Bean Tacos

Day 54:

Breakfast: Pineapple Kale Smoothie

Lunch: Sweet Potato and Spinach Curry

Dinner: Quinoa and Black Bean Salad

Day 55:

Breakfast: Tempeh Scramble

Lunch: Turkey and Veggie Stir Fry

Dinner: Grilled Salmon with Asparagus

Day 56:

Breakfast: Strawberry Banana Oatmeal

Lunch: Veggie-Packed Lentil Soup

Dinner: Pineapple & Tofu Stir-fry

Day 57:

Breakfast: Pineapple Spinach Smoothie

Lunch: Shrimp and Broccoli Stir Fry

Dinner: Shrimp Avocado Salad

Day 58:

Breakfast: Chia Berry Yogurt Parfait

Lunch: Butternut Squash Soup

Dinner: Chicken & Broccoli Stir-fry

Day 59:

Breakfast: Veggie Omelet
Lunch: Grilled Chicken and Veggie Skewers
Dinner: Garlic Shrimp with Zucchini Noodles

Day 60:

Breakfast: Almond Butter Toast with Blueberries
Lunch: Lentil Stew
Dinner: Mediterranean Bulgur Salad

Conclusion

Thank you for taking the time to read this book. Inflammation is a frequent condition characterized by symptoms such as pain, redness, and swelling. Inflammation is also a response to tissue damage or rejection. Avoid activities that induce inflammation and, if required, use a mixture of anti-inflammatory medicines to help lessen the symptoms of inflammation. Inflammation is not only uncomfortable, but it may also lead to major problems such as diabetes and heart disease in those who are unable to treat it alone with medicine. Poor food, injury, stress, certain drugs, and cigarette smoking can all contribute to inflammation.

It is vital to pay close attention to any signals your body sends you and not become disheartened if you do not experience instant benefits. However, it might take a long time for the body to naturally recover and restore equilibrium.

It is also crucial to keep in mind that many other variables can contribute to inflammation in the body, and that these might differ from person to person (for example, stress, depression, and anxiety). This is why it's vital for you to pay close attention to your own body by taking frequent measurements so you know what works and what doesn't.

The most essential thing to remember is to pay attention to your body rather than your intellect. Finally, bear in mind that a variety of things can trigger inflammation in the body, so any changes in your daily routine should be well monitored. If you observe any substantial changes, you may need to seek the help of someone who has more knowledge with natural therapies to enhance your health.

Thank you for making it this far. I've spent a long time drafting this work, and now I'd want to ask for your assistance in popularizing it. This would mean so much to me; it would bring me great joy to receive a nice review from you on Amazon; your reviews are far more essential than you realize!

INDEX

Printed in Great Britain
by Amazon

28463983R00053